Gastroenterology

Paul J. Thuluvath, MD, FRCP

Director of Hepatology
The Johns Hopkins Hospital
The Johns Hopkins University School of Medicine
Baltimore, Maryland

Anurag Maheshwari, MD

Gastroenterology Fellow
The Johns Hopkins Hospital
The Johns Hopkins University School of Medicine
Baltimore, Maryland

UK edition authors
Christopher Fox, Martin Lombard, and Emma Lam

UK series editor
Daniel Horton-Szar

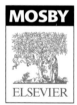

MOSBY

ELSEVIER

MOSBY
ELSEVIER

1600 John F. Kennedy Boulevard
Suite 1800
Philadelphia, PA 19103-2899

CRASH COURSE: GASTROENTEROLOGY

ISBN-13: 978-1-4160-2992-2

Copyright © 2006 by Mosby, Inc., an affiliate of Elsevier Inc.

ISBN-10: 1-4160-2992-3

Notice

Knowledge and best practice in this field are constantly changing. As new research and experience broaden our knowledge, changes in practice, treatment, and drug therapy may become necessary or appropriate. Readers are advised to check the most current information provided (i) on procedures featured or (ii) by the manufacturer of each product to be administered, to verify the recommended dose or formula, the method and duration of administration, and contraindications. It is the responsibility of the practitioner, relying on his or her own experience and knowledge of the patient, to make diagnoses, to determine dosages and the best treatment for each individual patient, and to take all appropriate safety precautions. To the fullest extent of the law, neither the Publisher nor the Editors assume any liability for any injury and/or damage to persons or property arising out or related to any use of the material contained in this book.

Adapted from Crash Course Gastrointestinal System 2e by Melanie Sarah Long, ISBN 0-7234-3251-1, © 2002, Elsevier Science Limited. All rights reserved.

The rights of Melanie Sarah Long to be identified as the author of this work have been asserted by her in accordance with the Copyright Designs and Patents Act, 1988.

Library of Congress Cataloging-in-Publication Data

Thuluvath, Paul J.
  Gastroenterology/Paul J. Thuluvath, Anurag Maheswari.—1st American ed.
    p. ; cm.—(Crash course)
  Includes index.
  ISBN 1-4160-2992-3
  1. Gastroenterology. 2. Digestive organs—Diseases. I. Maheswari, Anurag.
  II. Title. III. Series.
  [DNLM: 1. Gastrointestinal Diseases. WI 140 T534g 2006]
  RC801.T76 2006
  616.3'3—dc22   2005057652

Commissioning Editor: Alex Stibbe
Developmental Editor: Stan Ward
Project Manager: David Saltzberg
Design: Andy Chapman
Cover Design: Antbits Illustration
Illustration Manager: Mick Ruddy

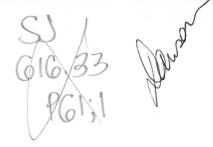

Working together to grow
libraries in developing countries

www.elsevier.com | www.bookaid.org | www.sabre.org

ELSEVIER   BOOK AID International   Sabre Foundation

Printed in China.

Last digit is the print number:
9 8 7 6 5 4 3 2 1

Preface

Crash Course: Gastroenterology is written primarily for students, residents, fellows, nurses, physician assistants, and nurse practitioners who want to learn the fundamentals of gastrointestinal and liver diseases in an easy manner.

The book will give a firm grounding for anyone who wants to master in gastroenterology and hepatology. It is not meant to be a reference text book; however, it provides a concise summary of our current understanding of the most salient aspects of the gastrointestinal and hepatic systems and offers an overview of common disorders and diagnoses. Important points are provided in a bulleted or pictorial format, which makes the book enjoyable to read. Care has been taken to cover all important areas.

We would appreciate your feedback as a reader so that we can continue to improve this series.

Paul J. Thuluvath, MD, FRCP

Contents

THE PATIENT PRESENTS WITH...

"Indigestion" encompasses a vast number of symptoms representing upper digestive tract problems with which a patient may present. These include:

- Heartburn.
- Fullness.
- Early satiety.
- Upper abdominal pain or ache.
- Flatulence.
- Hiccups.
- Belching.

The generic term that is useful to describe this constellation of symptoms is "dyspepsia":

- Prevalence of dyspepsia for the U.S. population is between 13% and 40% of the adult population. At least half of these seek advice from their family doctor.
- Dyspepsia accounts for 40% of referrals to gastroenterology clinics.

Dysphagia, or difficulty in swallowing, is dealt with separately.

History of the patient with indigestion

When taking a history from a patient with dyspepsia, it is useful to classify the problem according to the group of symptoms present, although this does not always correlate with the pathology. Dyspepsia is characterized as:

- "Reflux-like," if heartburn or chest pain predominates.
- "Ulcer-like," if the characteristics convey the impression of peptic ulcer disease. Upper gastrointestinal (GI) endoscopy (i.e., esophagogastroduodenoscopy) in these patients may be helpful to distinguish them from other conditions that mimic ulcer disease.

History of heartburn

Heartburn is the key to differentiating reflux-like dyspepsia from other forms. It is described as a burning sensation that the patient locates retrosternally (i.e., behind the sternum). It is a diffuse and poorly localized sensation, typically worse when the patient is lying and leaning forward. Rarely, reflux-related esophageal spasm may result in severe epigastric pain or intermittent dysphagia. Other symptoms that may be associated with reflux disease are wheezing or hoarseness of voice.

Excess saliva

"Waterbrash" is a specific phenomenon that the patient often describes as a flood of saliva in the mouth. Excess saliva is produced in the mouth and pharynx as a reflex response to acid in the lower esophagus.

Chest pain

This is a common feature of gastroesophageal reflux.

Pain due to heartburn often radiates between the shoulder blades. Esophageal spasm more commonly causes chest pain, which occurs after a meal but can arise spontaneously. The pain is:

- Typically felt behind the sternum.
- Often severe.
- Sometimes described as "something squeezing my inside."

Unlike cardiac pain, esophageal spasm tends not to be provoked by exertion. However, radiation of the pain to the jaw and left shoulder/arm can occur in severe cases. Exacerbation of the pain by changes in body position can be a helpful clue because reflux symptoms are worse when lying flat or stooping forward and are often relieved by adopting an upright posture. Nausea and vomiting are uncommon with reflux but can accompany myocardial infarction.

This pain is often confused with cardiac chest pain and, rather misleadingly, nitrates will relieve both spasm and angina, making it a diagnostic conundrum.

Common causes of esophageal spasm are:

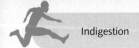

- Underlying acid reflux.
- Achalasia.

A history of either condition should raise suspicion in someone presenting with atypical chest pain.

Other causes of chest pain are usually easy to differentiate. Pain due to pulmonary disease (pleural inflammation) is more often sharp or stabbing "like a knife-cut" and is referred to as "pleuritic" pain. It is exacerbated by deep breaths and coughing, which do not affect pain of esophageal origin.

Nocturnal cough/asthma

Some patients with severe acid reflux do not complain of heartburn or chest pain but develop cough or hoarseness of voice or wheeze during the night when they are lying flat. They often lack symptoms during the daytime. Characteristically, they will demonstrate a "morning dip" in their peak-flow recordings (Fig. 1.1). The bronchospasm is thought to be due to microaspiration of acid, but a vagal reflex may also be involved because, experimentally, esophageal acid-induced bronchospasm is ablated by vagotomy.

Asthmatics have a higher than average prevalence of heartburn. Increased intra-abdominal pressure may play a role, but some drugs such as theophylline reduce the lower esophageal sphincter tone.

Aggravating and risk factors for reflux

The most important risk factor is increased intra-abdominal pressure (Fig. 1.2), which can "squeeze" the stomach contents upward and, ultimately, squeeze the stomach itself through the hiatus in the diaphragm (known as "hiatus hernia").

Discuss lifestyle habits and medication, including the following topics:

- Stooping and bending (occupation or sport) aggravate the problem.
- Spicy foods or those with a high fat content often aggravate the problem.
- Alcohol ingestion can result in increased acid secretion, delayed gastric emptying, and gastritis.
- Cigarettes often make reflux symptoms worse: nicotine causes smooth muscle relaxation in the lower esophageal sphincter.
- Nonsteroidal anti-inflammatory drug (NSAID) ingestion can interfere with prostaglandin cytoprotection.
- Caffeine and theophylline cause relaxation of the lower esophageal sphincter.

- Those drugs with an anticholinergic action can also lower esophageal tone (e.g., neuroleptics).

For most patients, antacids will provide some form of relief and are readily available as an over-the-counter medication.

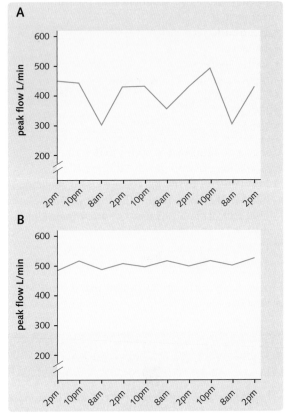

Fig. 1.1 A. Peak-flow measurement in an asthmatic patient demonstrating morning dip due to acid reflux. B. This was ablated when the patient took antisecretory medication before going to bed.

Risk factors for gastroesophageal reflux (GERD)
increased intra-abdominal pressures • sport (e.g., weight lifting) • occupation (e.g., stooping) • asthma • obesity • pregnancy drugs • alcohol • cigarette smoking • caffeine • anticholinergics

Fig. 1.2 Risk factors for gastroesophageal reflux.

All of these dyspeptic symptoms constitute gastroesophageal reflux disease (GERD).

A long history of heartburn followed by difficulty in swallowing (i.e., dysphagia) with improvement in the heartburn may herald a fibrotic stricture in the lower esophagus.

Epigastric pain

Epigastric pain is not a feature of GERD but characterizes dyspepsia as ulcer-like. It is a very common presenting complaint, but:

- The history is often vague.
- Sometimes patients have difficulty ascribing the term "pain" to what they feel. The pain is often described as "gnawing" or a persistent dull ache.

Pain due to:

- Peptic ulcer disease is occasionally more easily localized. The patient may point to a spot with one finger, although this is not a reliable sign.
- A gastric ulcer is often worse immediately after eating.

Peptic ulcers associated with NSAID use are often painless and many times present with occult bleeding.

Duodenal ulcer pain is:

- Commonly relieved by antacids.
- Worse at night, or in the fasted state, so the patient will often eat or drink milk before going to bed at night.

A family history is common. Find out about lifestyle habits such as smoking and alcohol consumption; these are important because they may contribute to gastritis. Medications such as NSAIDs can also cause gastritis, erosions, and ulcers.

Epigastric pain presenting with weight loss may indicate gastric carcinoma and warrants urgent investigation.

Flatulence, belching, bloating, and early satiety

Symptoms such as flatulence, belching, bloating, and early satiety are characteristically more vague. The term "nonulcer dyspepsia" is used to account for symptoms that occur in the absence of demonstrable acid reflux, duodenal and gastric ulcer, duodenitis or gastritis.

Nonulcer dyspepsia and peptic ulcer pain can be difficult to differentiate from other causes of acute and chronic abdominal pain (see Chapters 3 and 4). Some nonulcer dyspepsia is thought to be due to abnormal motility or abnormal sensitivity of the upper GI structures to distention.

Examining the patient with indigestion

Physical examination is usually unrevealing in a patient with reflux disease or esophageal spasm.
Check for:

- Obesity or pregnancy—these may support a diagnosis of GERD.
- Chronic GI blood loss and signs of iron deficiency—these may be caused by ulceration of the esophageal mucosa and may indicate chronic severe acid reflux or alternative GI pathology.
- Tooth erosion by acid—this may be a sign of very severe reflux.

Cardiac pain can sometimes be very difficult to differentiate from the pain of GERD and associated spasm. Features that may predispose a patient to ischemic heart disease should be looked for, such as:

- Tar staining on the fingers.
- Obesity.
- Stigmata of hypercholesterolemia, such as xanthomas.

Tenderness on deep palpation may indicate that the patient has ulcer-like dyspepsia due to gastritis or ulcer disease. Careful examination is important to exclude other causes of abdominal pain.

Investigating indigestion

An algorithm for the evaluation of the patient with indigestion is shown in Fig. 1.3.

In the majority of cases of reflux the symptoms are mild, and the diagnosis can often be made

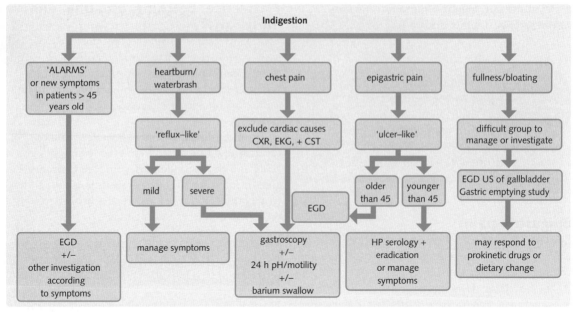

Fig. 1.3 Algorithm for the evaluation of patients with dyspepsia (CXR, chest X-ray; EKG, electrocardiography; CST, cardiac stress test; EGD, esophagogastroduodenoscopy; US, ultrasound; HP, *Helicobacter pylori*).

clinically and appropriate treatment commenced. More symptomatic cases may require investigation to exclude or confirm underlying esophagitis. Any ALARMS symptoms are an indication for urgent referral and investigation.

ALARMS symptoms in dyspepsia:
- **A**nemia.
- **L**oss of weight.
- **A**norexia.
- **R**efractory to antisecretory medication.
- **M**elena.
- **S**wallowing problems.

Persistent continuous vomiting should be added to this list.

Upper GI tract malignancy can also present with these symptoms; therefore, patients older than 45 years of age with recent onset of persisting, dyspeptic symptoms should usually undergo prompt endoscopy (upper GI tract cancer is exceptionally rare in persons younger than the age of 45 years except in the case of familial cancer syndromes).

Many practitioners now use *Helicobacter* serology in association with the symptom of dyspepsia to identify patients who may benefit from empirical eradication treatment for *Helicobacter* (see below).

Investigations to consider are discussed below.

Complete blood count

A complete blood count may be performed to exclude underlying anemia. Microcytic anemia is common with severe esophagitis but rare in peptic ulcer disease. Plummer-Vinson syndrome comprises iron deficiency anemia associated with an esophageal web. A high platelet count can indicate chronic GI bleeding.

Electrocardiography

Electrocardiography is particularly useful for patients with atypical-sounding pain that may be due to esophageal spasm or angina pectoris. However, nonspecific T-wave changes can occur with reflux. An exercise tolerance test may be necessary to differentiate between esophageal and cardiac pain.

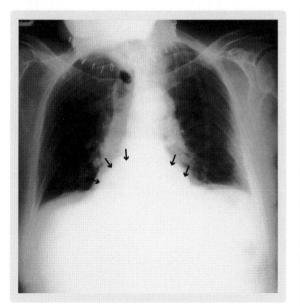

Fig. 1.4 Chest X-ray showing a hiatus hernia (arrows) behind the cardiac shadow. (Incidentally shown on this X-ray are surgical staples around the neck following operative dissection.)

Occasionally, other investigations such as a thallium scan and coronary angiography are necessary to discriminate between cardiac and esophageal symptoms.

Chest X-ray

A chest X-ray may demonstrate a hiatus hernia behind the cardiac shadow (Fig. 1.4).

Barium study

Cine esophagogram and upper GI tract series or scintigraphy are useful in demonstrating reflux. This can give rise to a "corkscrew" appearance during an attack of spasm and is usually diagnostic (Fig. 1.5).

Esophageal motility studies

Esophageal motility studies may be required to demonstrate diffuse contraction and reduced peristalsis during a provoked attack. Pressures in the esophagus can be exceedingly high, and the term "nutcracker esophagus" has been coined for these cases.

pH monitoring

pH monitoring is usually reserved for patients whose symptoms are more marked than expected from the

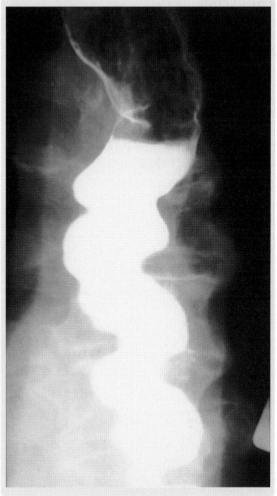

Fig. 1.5 Barium swallow demonstration of "corkscrew" esophagus caused by esophageal spasm.

endoscopic findings, or for those who are refractory to medical treatment.

Breath tests

Breath tests have been devised to detect the presence of *Helicobacter pylori* without the requirement of endoscopy and biopsy (see Chapter 24).

Serology

Serology can be used to identify past infection with *H. pylori*. However, the immunoglobulin G antibody test gives no indication of the current state of infection and is not useful for assessing response to treatment.

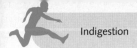

Endoscopy

Endoscopy is useful for the assessment of the presence, extent, and severity of esophagitis. It can also be used to identify:

- Hiatal hernia—this may be noted on endoscopy but itself is not diagnostic of acid reflux because it is often an incidental finding, especially in elderly people.
- Ulcer disease and gastritis—biopsy specimens can be taken to differentiate each type, to exclude malignancy, and to look for the presence of *H. pylori*.

Barium meal

Barium meal is an alternative for patients for whom endoscopy may be difficult. It may demonstrate ulcer disease or malignancy.

Gastric emptying studies

Scintigraphy (nuclear medicine) for both solid and liquid gastric emptying may help in the investigation of gastric motility disorders.

Differential diagnosis

The patient will usually complain of difficulty swallowing or the sensation of food sticking as it goes down (i.e., dysphagia). Difficulty with the passage of food typically begins with solids like bread or meat, followed by liquids if the condition is progressive. The condition is usually painless and is due to a narrowing of the esophageal lumen.

The differential diagnosis includes, in order of importance, the following:
- Esophageal carcinoma.
- Achalasia.
- Benign esophageal stricture.
- Esophagitis.
- Esophageal spasm.
- Failure of peristalsis due to other reasons (e.g., scleroderma).
- Esophageal pouch or diverticulum.
- Esophageal web.
- Incarcerated hiatus hernia.
- Foreign body obstruction.

 Dysphagia is often unnoticed or even denied by patients until it becomes troublesome. They may relieve their distress by changing posture, belching, regurgitating food, or taking a drink.

History of the patient with swallowing problems

Taking a careful history of the presenting complaint is the key to sorting out the differential diagnosis. Important features to ask about are discussed below.

Duration of symptoms
A long or intermittent history, usually accompanied by maneuvers to relieve the symptoms, often indicates anatomic or mechanical obstruction due to:

- Pouch.
- Diverticulum.
- Webs.
- Incarcerated hernia.

The first three are more common in younger adults, the last in elderly people.

Level at which dysphagia occurs
The level of dysphagia is poorly localized in most cases. Attempt to determine the level at which dysphagia is experienced:
- High-level dysphagia can be due to cricopharyngeal spasm, a contraction of the cricopharyngeus muscle and inferior constrictors that is closely associated with pharyngeal pouch syndrome.
- Low-level dysphagia is more common with peptic strictures.
- Carcinoma occurs at all levels (Fig. 2.1).

 The patient's perception of the level at which dysphagia occurs is not a reliable indication of the level of obstruction.

Weight loss
Minor weight loss is common because patients may have modified their diets to cope with dysphagia. Significant weight loss is an ominous sign and almost always indicates carcinoma.

History of heartburn
A history of heartburn preceding the dysphagia is highly suggestive of benign esophageal stricture, which often prevents further reflux.

Reflux
Reflux and dysphagia occurring together suggest achalasia, a condition in which there is uncoordinated esophageal peristalsis and failure to relax the lower

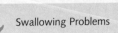
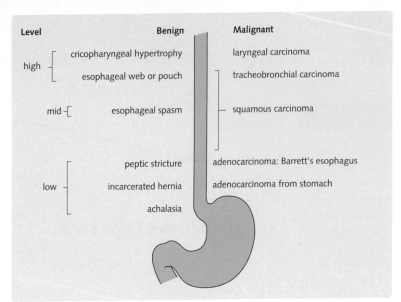

Level	Benign	Malignant
high	cricopharyngeal hypertrophy esophageal web or pouch	laryngeal carcinoma tracheobronchial carcinoma
mid	esophageal spasm	squamous carcinoma
low	peptic stricture incarcerated hernia achalasia	adenocarcinoma: Barrett's esophagus adenocarcinoma from stomach

Fig. 2.1 Sites at which esophageal lesions cause dysphagia. The patient will often describe the level of obstruction as high, mid, or lower chest, but this does not reliably correlate with the site or nature of pathology.

esophageal sphincter. This tends to present in early adulthood with chest pain occurring due to esophageal spasm, which can be mistaken for cardiac pain.

Regurgitation of food

Regurgitation of food is common if pouches are present. It differs from vomiting in that:

- There is an absence of nausea.
- Only small boluses are regurgitated back into the mouth and are often swallowed immediately.

Fluids are often more problematic than solids. Occasionally, dysphagia may be present because of obstruction by the pouch itself, but this is usually intermittent.

Regurgitation is not a feature of esophageal carcinoma or benign strictures.

Recurrent pulmonary infections

Recurrent pulmonary infections resulting from aspiration can be due to:

- Achalasia.
- Pouches.
- Diverticula.

Progression of dysphagia

Progressive dysphagia is manifest by the patient finding increasing difficulty with soft foods or liquids, following difficulty with solids. This may occur over a relatively short duration (weeks or months) and is an ominous development, most often signifying an esophageal carcinoma.

Pain with dysphagia

Pain on swallowing is termed "odynophagia" and may or may not be accompanied by dysphagia. Odynophagia may be caused by:

- Infection with *Candida* species. This is the most common cause and may result from underlying immunosuppression (e.g., corticosteroids or other immunosuppressive treatments, diabetes, malignancy, or immunodeficiency). Herpes and cytomegalovirus infection of the esophagus are more likely to be found in people infected with HIV.
- Impaction of a foreign body. This may cause dysphagia and will usually have an obvious history (e.g., fish bones represent the most common cause).

Esophageal candidiasis should always prompt the clinician to look for underlying immunosuppression.

Pain between the shoulder blades in association with heartburn usually signifies esophagitis.

A "lump" in the throat can be due to pharyngitis but is also a presentation of globus hystericus. Globus is a functional disorder that usually affects young females. True dysphagia of solids followed by difficulty with liquids is absent. A history suggestive of depression and/or anxiety can often be elicited, and it is important to establish the root of the patient's concern to allay unfounded fears (e.g., "My father died of throat cancer").

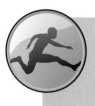 The diagnosis of globus should not be accepted without investigation and exclusion of more common or more sinister causes of dysphagia.

Important past medical history

Find out about the patient's past medical history, particularly:

- Risk factors for carcinoma. These include Barrett's esophagitis, tylosis, and smoking.
- Chronic systemic diseases. Neuromuscular disorders such as motor neuron disease, myasthenia gravis, and mytonia dystrophica are associated with disordered peristalsis.
- Collagen vascular disease (e.g., scleroderma), which can interfere with the elasticity of the esophagus and impair peristalsis.

Examining the patient with swallowing problems

Look out for:
- Weight loss. If marked, this should give cause for concern; patients with carcinoma are often cachectic. A healthy, well-nourished patient with a history of dysphagia usually indicates a benign etiology, but not exclusively so.
- Anemia. Sometimes clinically evident, anemia can occur with esophagitis and classically has been a feature associated with esophageal web (e.g., Plummer-Vinson or Paterson-Kelly syndrome). It is more common with malignant disease.
- Systemic features such as clubbing, tylosis (i.e., thickening of the palms of the hand and soles of the feet), supraclavicular lymph nodes, and hepatomegaly. These are suggestive of malignant disease in the context of dysphagia.
- An epigastric mass. This may be palpable if the tumor extends into the cardia and certainly signifies extensive disease. However, there are no clinical signs that are specific for esophageal carcinoma.

Investigating swallowing problems

It is imperative to evaluate any patient who presents with dysphagia. A summary algorithm is shown in Fig. 2.2.

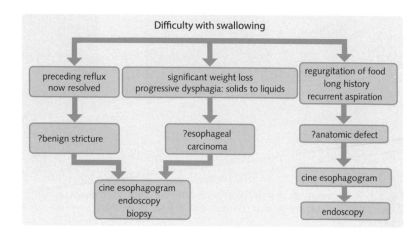

Fig. 2.2 Algorithm for the evaluation of a patient with difficulty in swallowing.

Complete blood count and biochemistry

Full blood count and biochemistry should be performed to assess anemia and, in severe cases, dehydration. Blood tests such as serum glucose and thyroid function will exclude other causes of weight loss such as diabetes and thyrotoxicosis. Occasionally, a retrosternal goiter may cause dysphagia. Liver biochemistry and calcium levels may be deranged in cases of advanced malignancy.

An imaging study of the esophagus should precede endoscopic evaluation in cases of dysphagia.

Endoscopy

Endoscopy is the method of investigation of choice for most patients with a history of dysphagia because, in addition to directly visualizing the esophageal mucosa, biopsies can be undertaken to allow histologic differentiation of benign and malignant lesions.

Laryngoscopy

Laryngoscopy may be necessary to investigate high causes of dysphagia.

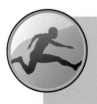

When endoscopy is unrevealing and dysphagia persists or is high level, a cine esophagogram should always be performed as well.

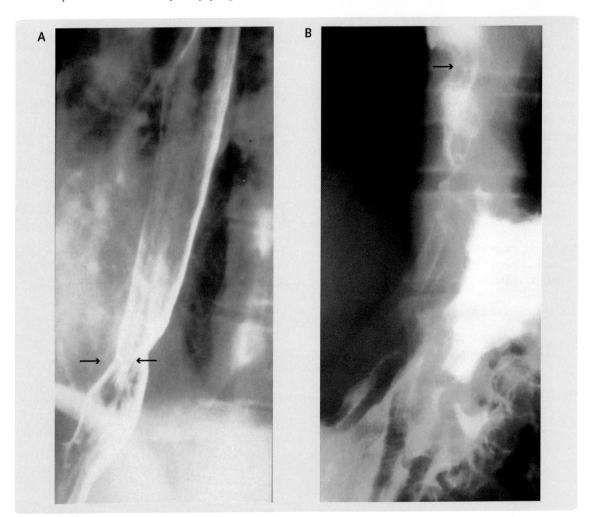

Fig. 2.3 A. Barium swallow showing smooth tapering stricture of benign esophageal type (arrows). B. The ''shouldered'' appearance of malignant stricture (arrow) due to infiltration of the esophagus from adenocarcinoma of the stomach cardia.

Cine esophagogram

Cine esophagogram can be undertaken for patients who are unable to tolerate endoscopy, but appearances between benign and malignant strictures can be difficult to interpret. Generally:

- Benign strictures are smooth and tapering.
- Malignant strictures are irregular and "shouldered" (Fig. 2.3).
- Barium study is very useful in demonstrating anatomic anomalies such as:
  - Pouches, usually high in the midline, caused by a defect in the overlapping muscle layers.
  - Diverticula, usually small and associated with disordered peristalsis.
  - Webs, which can be high at the cricopharyngeus or lower down the esophagus.
  - A Schatzki ring, which is a fibromuscular attachment originating from the diaphragm. This anomaly is usually associated with a small hiatus hernia.

Barium study can be diagnostic of achalasia with the typical appearance of:

- A dilated esophagus with no peristalsis.
- A narrowed lower esophagus (bird's beak appearance) due to the failure of the lower esophageal sphincter to relax (see Fig. 14.6).

Achalasia is often missed at endoscopy.

Esophageal motility studies

Esophageal motility studies are useful to confirm spasm or achalasia. Twenty-four–hour esophageal pH monitoring is useful to confirm acid reflux (see Figs. 24.9 and 24.10).

Chest X-ray

A chest X-ray, often forgotten, provides useful information about patients with swallowing problems, especially those who present with pneumonia. A dilated esophagus can be seen as a double cardiac shadow with a fluid level behind the heart.

Other investigations

Occasionally, the cause of dysphagia may be difficult to find.

Bronchoscopy or a computed tomography scan may be required if tracheobronchial carcinoma is suspected.

Patients found to have a malignant stricture will need to be assessed for surgical resection. Gross metastatic spread can be identified by ultrasound of the liver or computed tomography scan of the thorax. For locoregional spread, endoscopic ultrasound is the best single staging test.

Electrocardiography

All patients who present with chest or abdominal pain should undergo an electrocardiogram to exclude myocardial infarction (Fig. 3.3). Some T-wave changes are nonspecific and can be seen in many causes of acute abdominal pain, although ultimately cardiac enzyme levels may need to be measured to exclude myocardial injury.

Endoscopy

Esophagogastroduodenoscopy may be indicated if peptic ulcer disease is suspected but would be contraindicated in many causes of acute abdominal pain (e.g., perforation).

Urgent endoscopic retrograde cholangiopancreatography may be indicated for suspected gallstone pancreatitis or acute cholangitis.

This would usually follow ultrasound examination or computed tomography scan.

In both conditions, emergency sphincterotomy and stone removal is very effective in patients with bile duct stones and also may be beneficial in patients with moderate to severe pancreatitis.

Surgery

Many of the causes of acute abdominal pain are surgical emergencies. Occasionally, no cause is apparent and diagnostic laparotomy or laparoscopy can be useful in these situations (e.g., peritonitis of uncertain cause).

Summary

An algorithm summarizing the investigation of acute abdominal pain is shown in Fig. 3.4.

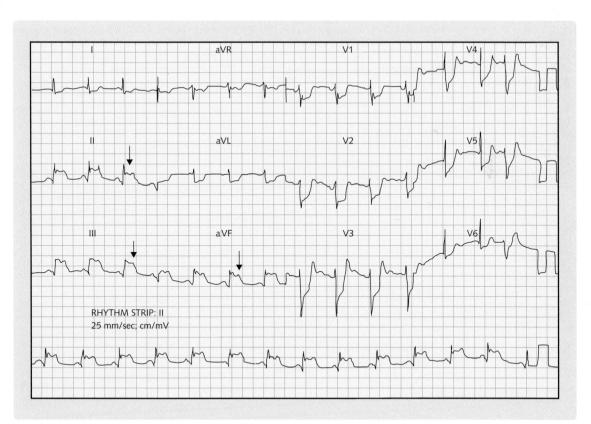

Fig. 3.3 Electrocardiogram from a patient presenting with acute abdominal pain. ST segment elevation in leads II, III, and aVF (arrows) supports a diagnosis of inferior myocardial infarction (aVR, unipolar limb lead on the right arm; aVL, unipolar limb lead on the left arm; aVF, augmented unipolar limb leads).

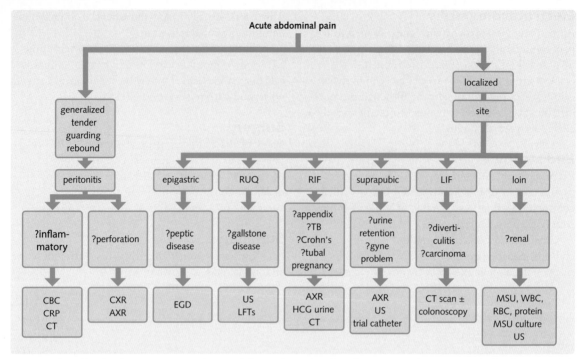

Fig. 3.4 Algorithm for the investigation of acute abdominal pain (RUQ, right upper quadrant; RIF, right iliac fossa; LIF, left iliac fossa; TB, tuberculosis; gyne, gynecologic; CBC, complete blood cell count; CRP, C-reactive protein; CT, computed tomography; CXR, chest X-ray; AXR, abdominal X-ray; EGD, esophagogastroduodenoscopy; US, ultrasound; LFTs, liver function tests; HCG, human chorionic gonadotropin [pregnancy test)]; MSU, midstream urine; WBC, white blood cells; RBC, red blood cells).

4. Chronic Abdominal Pain

Chronic abdominal pain is a common complaint that accounts for about 40% of referral to gastroenterology outpatient clinics. The symptoms are often of an intermittent nature, with pain-free periods in between. The list of differential diagnoses is vast, and only those commonly seen in clinical practice are discussed here. There is considerable overlap between some of these symptoms and "indigestion" discussed in Chapter 1, but pain is not really a prominent symptom in dyspepsia and is discussed in more detail here.

The common differential diagnoses for chronic abdominal pain include:
- Peptic ulcer disease.
- Chronic pancreatitis.
- Chronic cholecystitis.
- Chronic appendicitis.
- Irritable bowel syndrome.
- Constipation.
- Subacute bowel obstruction.
- Crohn's disease.
- Intestinal malignancy.
- Mesenteric ischemia.
- Gynecologic causes (e.g., endometriosis, pelvic inflammatory disease).
- Gastroparesis.

History of the patient with chronic abdominal pain

As with acute abdominal pain, a detailed patient history is essential to focus the differential diagnosis. Several important features need to be discovered, and these are discussed below.

Site and radiation of the pain
The most obvious clue to the etiology is the site of the pain and its radiation.

Chronic pain in the upper abdomen is suggestive of:
- Peptic ulcer disease.
- Chronic cholecystitis.
- Chronic pancreatitis.

Pain at particular sites may be even more specific:
- Pain in the right upper quadrant is commonly of liver or biliary origin.
- Pain in the right iliac fossa may suggest Crohn's disease (i.e., terminal ileal disease).
- Pain in the loin may be due to chronic pyelonephritis.
- Pain in the lower abdomen is usually due to colonic or gynecologic problems.

Character
The character of chronic pain is often vague, but certain features are helpful.
- Most chronic abdominal pain is described as a dull ache, which is suggestive of visceral peritoneal involvement (e.g., chronic pancreatitis, intestinal malignancy, gynecologic causes).
- Sharp, stabbing, or colicky pain may be associated with distention of a viscus (e.g., biliary colic, constipation, or irritable bowel syndrome).

Take a history of each episode of pain. Has hospital admission been necessary? Evaluation of old medical notes can be very revealing.

Exacerbating and relieving factors
Identification of exacerbating and relieving factors is sometimes helpful. The patient may have had the pain for some time and may have experimented with ways to relieve or exacerbate the pain, such as with food or alcohol.

Food can have the following effects:
- It may aggravate biliary causes, characteristically occurring 20 to 30 minutes after a meal, and there may be fat intolerance, although this is not specific for a particular diagnosis.
- With mesenteric ischemia (also known as "abdominal angina"), the patient may notice that pain occurs 1 to 2 hours after food intake, and this results in a reluctance to eat for fear of pain.
- It can relieve the pain of a duodenal ulcer, particularly if the patient drinks milk at bedtime.

Alcohol:
- Worsens chronic pancreatitis and gastritis, but the patient does not always modify his or her behavior.

Defecation or passage of flatus:
- Relieves lower abdominal pain due to constipation or irritable bowel.
- May exacerbate pain due to local inflammatory conditions of the anus or rectum, or in cases of obstruction.

Menstruation:
- Painful periods should be obvious, but ectopic areas of endometriosis may also induce pain at the time of menstruation.
- Pain in mid cycle can occur with ovulation (i.e., mittelschmerz) or occasionally with the occurrence of ovarian cysts.

Associated features

Patients may not notice other symptoms or realize their significance in relation to the pain. It is therefore important to ask specifically about:
- Distention or bloating. If intermittent, this is suggestive of irritable bowel syndrome or subacute obstruction; if progressive, it may indicate development of a mass or ascites.
- Weight loss. Think of underlying malignancy (e.g., pancreatic or intestinal), especially in elderly patients. In younger patients, think of Crohn's disease or lymphoma. Weight loss may also result from avoidance of food.
- Change in bowel habit. Alternating constipation or diarrhea may be due to a change in diet, but intestinal malignancy must be excluded in patients older than 45 years.
- Rectal bleeding. This may signify an underlying inflammatory or malignant process (see Chapter 10).
- Vaginal discharge. Pelvic inflammatory disease is something the patient may be embarrassed to volunteer information about.

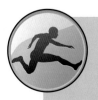

Many patients will be reluctant to reveal their level of alcohol consumption. Careful questioning is often required! Try to ascertain their habits from several angles.

Examining the patient with chronic abdominal pain

On general inspection, important features to note include:
- Obvious signs of weight loss.
- Pigmentation, pallor, or jaundice.
- Signs of dehydration.

In the neck, look for:
- Lymphadenopathy, particularly in the supraclavicular regions.
- Goiter.

Abdominal inspection and palpation may reveal:
- Scars from previous surgery. Patients occasionally omit information about previous operations.
- Distention. Is it uniform due to ascites or asymmetrical due to a mass?
- Peristalsis. This may be obvious in thin people with intestinal obstruction.
- A mass. Its anatomic location usually indicates the etiology (e.g., epigastric in gastric malignancy, right iliac fossa in Crohn's disease, or an appendix mass).
- Stigmata of chronic alcohol misuse (e.g., spider nevi, umbilical varices, and other signs of chronic liver disease).

Other features to note are:
- Signs of peripheral vascular disease, which may accompany mesenteric ischemia.
- Tenderness in the fornix or vaginal discharge, suggesting pelvic inflammatory disease.
- Rectal examination should always be performed for patients with lower abdominal pain.

Investigating chronic abdominal pain

Complete blood count

Anemia may be due to blood loss giving rise to a microcytic hypochromic picture of iron deficiency. In malignant or inflammatory disease, a normocytic anemia may also occur. A raised white blood cell count is indicative of underlying infection or inflammation. Platelet levels can be raised in chronic inflammatory disease or chronic gastrointestinal blood loss.

Iron deficiency anemia in the context of chronic abdominal pain should always prompt endosopic examination of both the upper and lower gastrointestinal tract.

Biochemistry

Often a range of biochemistry tests is undertaken as a routine, but it is essential to interpret these in the clinical context. The following may be helpful:

- Electrolyte levels can be disturbed if diarrhea or vomiting had occurred (e.g., low potassium).
- Calcium levels can be raised in malignant disease, but hypercalcemia for other reasons (e.g., hyperparathyroidism) may also cause chronic abdominal pain.
- Amylase levels can be raised slightly and nonspecifically with many causes of abdominal pain. This is normal in chronic pancreatitis, in contradistinction to acute pancreatitis.
- Liver enzyme abnormalities are common with cholangitis or gallstone problems.
- Urea levels may be raised if dehydration is present or low if the patient has been anorectic, has malabsorption, or has liver disease.

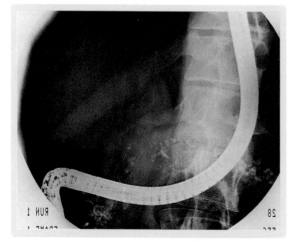

Fig. 4.1 Abdominal calcification is seen across the pancreatic area in a preinjection endoscopic retrograde cholangiopancreatogram.

- A thyroid function test should be performed because hypothyroidism is an occasional cause of abdominal pain.
- Tumor markers such as CEA or CA19.9 may be useful but need to be interpreted with caution.

Radiology

Although often unrevealing, a plain abdominal radiograph may reveal:

- Calcification indicative of chronic pancreatitis, gallstones, or aortic aneurysm (Fig. 4.1).
- Fecal loading suggestive of chronic constipation.
- Dilated bowel indicative of subacute obstruction.

Abdominal ultrasound is useful to identify:

- Gallstones causing chronic cholecystitis or bile duct obstruction.
- Liver metastases, which commonly arise from the colon or breast (Fig. 4.2).
- Chronic pancreatitis or carcinoma of the body of pancreas.

In the case of intra-abdominal lymphadenopathy, suggesting lymphoma or metastatic disease, contrast studies can be helpful.

- Small bowel barium studies would help identify terminal ileal strictures due to Crohn's disease.
- Large bowel barium enema is used to confirm diverticular disease or exclude colonic carcinoma.

Computed tomography of the abdomen may be required to visualize chronic pancreatitis or pancreatic carcinoma and to search for, or stage, lymphoma.

Endoscopy

Esophagogastroduodenoscopy is useful to investigate dyspepsia (see Chapter 1) and to exclude gastric carcinoma from the differential diagnosis. Colonoscopy may be required to confirm diverticular disease or to exclude colonic carcinoma.

Surgery

Despite extensive (and sometimes expensive!) investigation, in some cases no cause for chronic abdominal pain may be found. In these situations, and after careful consideration, a diagnostic laparoscopy can be useful (e.g., to identify endometriosis).

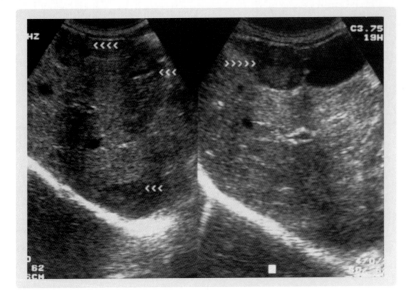

Fig. 4.2 Ultrasound scan showing multiple areas of different echogenicity and size in the liver, suggestive of metastases.

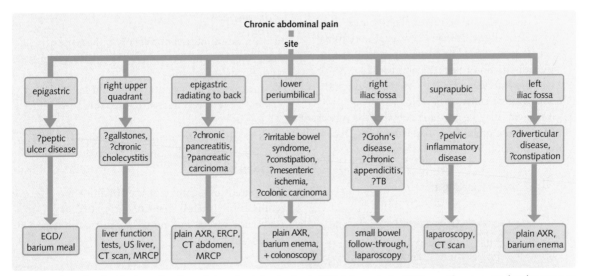

Fig. 4.3 Algorithm for the investigation of chronic abdominal pain (TB, tuberculosis; EGD, esophagogastroduodenoscopy; US, ultrasound; CT, computed tomography; MRCP, magnetic resonance cholangiopancreatography; AXR, abdominal X-ray; ERCP, endoscopic retrograde cholangiopancreatography).

Summary

An algorithm summarizing the investigation of chronic abdominal pain is shown in Fig. 4.3.

Abdominal examination is necessary to establish whether there is any evidence of intestinal obstruction and to identify any masses that may be responsible.

A succussion splash may be present with gastric outlet obstruction.

Investigating vomiting problems

Investigation may be necessary both to identify the cause of vomiting and to monitor its metabolic effects.

Blood tests

Consider the following blood tests:

- Complete blood count may support an impression of dehydration if the hematocrit level is high. Raised white blood cell count can indicate infection.
- The blood urea level is mildly raised in dehydration, but higher levels may be indicative of renal failure or upper GI tract bleeding, both of which can cause vomiting.
- The blood glucose level is high in diabetic ketoacidosis.

- Hyperkalemia with hyponatremia may suggest adrenal insufficiency. Persistent vomiting will also cause hypokalemic alkalosis (i.e., low potassium with elevated bicarbonate).
- Hypercalcemia from any cause can present with vomiting.
- Liver enzyme levels may reveal a pattern of acute hepatitis, which sometimes presents with vomiting.

Microbiologic tests

Blood culture tests and cerebrospinal fluid tap may be indicated if the patient is very ill or if meningitis is suspected.

Radiology

Plain abdominal X-ray is useful to exclude obstruction (e.g., due to pyloric stenosis).

A computed tomography scan of the head may be indicated by the clinical picture.

Summary

An algorithm summarizing the investigation of vomiting is shown in Fig. 7.1.

8. Hematemesis and Melena

"Hematemesis" refers to the vomiting of blood. "Melena" is the passage of black, tarry, and foul-smelling stools resulting from the effect of the digestive process on fresh blood. Hematemesis and melena are usually caused by upper gastrointestinal (GI) tract bleeding.

Common causes include:
- Reflux esophagitis.
- Mallory-Weiss tear.
- Esophageal or gastric varices.
- Gastric ulcers or erosions.
- Gastric carcinoma.
- Duodenal ulceration.
- Hereditary telangiectasia.

 The effects of taking iron tablets can be confused with melena because these supplements produce dark or black stool. However, iron stools have a sticky or grainy consistency unlike the tarry, runny nature of melena. Melena also has a characteristic odor!

History of the patient with hematemesis

The first fact that needs to be established is whether a patient is experiencing true hematemesis.
- Hemoptysis is coughing of blood and can sometimes be confused with hematemesis.
- Epistaxis (i.e., nosebleed), especially if it is severe and the blood is often swallowed, can be difficult to differentiate from true hematemesis.
- Melena should always follow true hematemesis, but it must not be confused with bleeding from the colon or rectum, which produces dark or bright red blood, respectively.

There are a few clues to help to decide the cause of bleeding. These are discussed below.

Volume of blood loss

Try to estimate this in terms that the patient can understand (e.g., one half cup, 2 cups). Be aware that the amount of blood is often overestimated.
- A large hematemesis is indicative of a significant GI tract bleed and is more likely to be a result of bleeding from esophageal varices or an arterial bleed from peptic ulceration.
- A small bleed may manifest itself as altered blood if it has been present in the stomach for some time. The patient may complain of vomiting "coffee grounds."

Past medical history

Find out whether the patient suffers from chronic liver disease. Esophageal variceal hemorrhage, consequent on portal hypertension, is then more likely; however, these patients also get peptic ulcers.

There may be a personal or family history of recurrent GI tract bleeds due to hereditary hemorrhagic telangiectasia.

Drug history

When taking the patient's history, pay particular attention to use of nonsteroidal anti-inflammatory drugs, including low-dose aspirin. These drugs predispose to reflux esophagitis, gastritis, and gastric erosions, especially in elderly persons, causing both occult and manifest hemorrhage. Corticosteroid tablets (e.g., prednisone) increase this risk if administered concurrently.

Patients taking anticoagulants such as warfarin to treat such conditions as venous thromboses, atrial fibrillation, or prosthetic heart valves may have large hemorrhages from very minor gastric erosions.

Associated features

Vigorous vomiting or retching preceding the hematemesis is suggestive of a Mallory-Weiss tear of the mucosa across the gastroesophageal junction. This can result in significant hemorrhage, although it is usually self-limiting.

An antecedent history of upper abdominal pain is suggestive of peptic ulcer disease or gastritis.

Heartburn may be due to acid reflux causing reflux esophagitis.

Examining the patient with hematemesis

If the hemorrhage has been severe, it will be necessary to examine and resuscitate the patient concurrently, while trying to ascertain the cause. Important features to look for are:
- Hypotension—systolic blood pressure less than 100 mmHg (with or without alteration of consciousness).
- Tachycardia—heart rate greater than 100.
- Pallor.
- Cold, clammy peripheries.

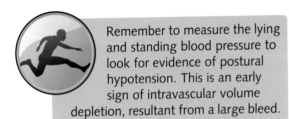

Remember to measure the lying and standing blood pressure to look for evidence of postural hypotension. This is an early sign of intravascular volume depletion, resultant from a large bleed.

Features of liver disease suggesting the presence of esophageal varices may be obvious:

- Jaundice.
- Parotitis.
- Spider nevi.
- Palmar erythema.
- Hepatosplenomegaly.
- Ascites.

Perioral telangiectasia may suggest hereditary hemorrhagic telangiectasia. A rectal examination is imperative to establish the presence of melena.

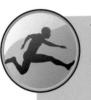

The top priority in managing hematemesis is to make sure you have adequate intravenous access to resuscitate the patient, even before you take a full history. The airway should always be protected.

Investigating hematemesis

Endoscopy is the definitive test for all GI tract bleeding. If hematemesis and melena are obvious or significant, urgent endoscopy is indicated to establish the cause and stop the bleeding. However, the patient should always be resuscitated first.

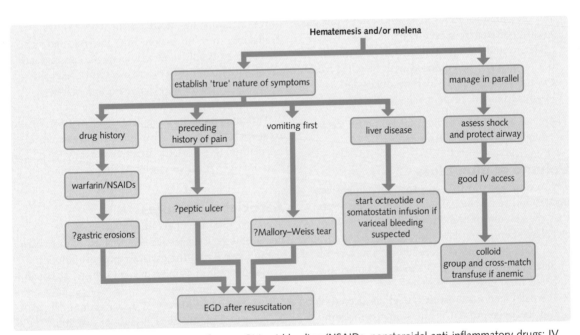

Fig. 8.1 Algorithm for the investigation of upper GI tract bleeding (NSAIDs, nonsteroidal anti-inflammatory drugs; IV, intravenous; EGD, esophagogastroduodenoscopy).

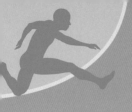

10. Rectal Bleeding

"Rectal bleeding" usually refers to bright red bleeding due to anorectal pathology. A clear, precise patient history will determine the site and the underlying cause in most cases.

Any rectal bleeding other than bright red blood indicates that the blood has been altered by bacterial or enzymatic digestion higher up in the colon or small bowel. The importance of distinguishing altered blood from bleeding that is solely occurring in the rectum cannot be overemphasized.

Causes of bright red rectal bleeding include:
- Hemorrhoids.
- Anal fissure.
- Anorectal carcinoma or polyps.
- Angiodysplasia.
- Diverticular disease.
- Inflammatory bowel disease.

History of the patient with rectal bleeding

Establish the relationship between the onset of rectal bleeding and passage of stool because this will give important clues about the etiology:
- "Spotting" of bright red blood appearing on toilet paper only after the passage of stool is highly suggestive of hemorrhoids or anal fissure if there is associated pain on defecation.
- Presence of blood that is separate from feces (often noticed as bright red fresh blood in the toilet pan) is associated with low rectal lesions such as hemorrhoids and anorectal carcinoma, where passage of mucus is also common. Pain is not usually a feature, except where anal fissure is also present with the hemorrhoids.
- Passage of dark red blood mixed in with the stool is suggestive of a high rectal lesion such as carcinoma, angiodysplasia, or an inflamed diverticulum.

Associated features such as weight loss, diarrhea, or abdominal pain suggest serious pathology rather than simple anorectal conditions.

Examining the patient with rectal bleeding

A general examination looking for evidence of anemia, cachexia, or lymphadenopathy is followed by an abdominal examination. Fecal masses may be palpable if there is significant constipation, which predisposes the patient to hemorrhoids and anal fissure. Left iliac fossa tenderness, with or without guarding, is suggestive of inflamed diverticula.
- Rectal examination is mandatory in this situation; take particular note of the external, perianal area. Anal tags suggest previously thrombosed hemorrhoids.
- Mucus discharge may be seen in inflammatory bowel disease and anorectal carcinoma.
- Increased anal tone and pain on rectal examination are highly indicative of anal fissure.
- Hard feces in the rectum may suggest chronic constipation or anal fissure.
- Masses due to rectal carcinoma or polyp can also be palpated on rectal examination.

Proctoscopy enables examination of the position of hemorrhoids, which may be treated with sclerotherapy. Anal fissures can also be seen, although it is unlikely that a patient with this painful condition will tolerate the passage of a proctoscope.

Rigid sigmoidoscopy can visualize up to 15 to 20 cm from the anal margin, and biopsy specimens can be taken of any suspicious lesion to detect carcinoma or inflammatory bowel disease.

Blood loss from hemorrhoids is usually not severe enough to cause anemia. Rectal bleeding with anemia is more likely to be due to carcinoma, angiodysplasia, or inflammatory bowel disease.

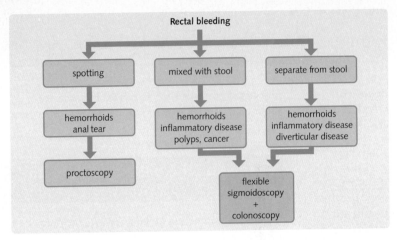

Fig. 10.1 Investigation of rectal bleeding.

Investigating rectal bleeding

The majority of conditions can be diagnosed with a careful history and examination with proctoscopy and sigmoidoscopy. However, further investigation may be required if the diagnosis is equivocal:

- Complete blood count is essential to establish whether anemia is present.
- Colonoscopy or flexible sigmoidoscopy allows higher sigmoid lesions and many vascular lesions, such as angiodysplasia, to be seen.

More than two thirds of all colonic polyps and tumors occur within 60 cm of the anal margin.
- Angiography can be performed to locate the site of bleeding from angiodysplasia. However, this is reserved for circumstances where there is a high index of suspicion and the patient has evidence of active bleeding.

Summary
An algorithm summarizing the investigation of rectal bleeding is shown in Fig. 10.1.

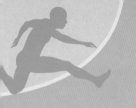

Anemia is a low hemoglobin concentration in plasma due to a low red cell mass. The symptoms of anemia occur as a result of the reduced oxygen-carrying capacity of blood and therefore the reduced delivery of oxygen to tissues. Gastrointestinal causes of anemia include:

- Reduced intake (e.g., dietary deficiencies of iron, folate, and vitamin B_{12}).
- Reduced absorption (e.g., pernicious anemia, small bowel disease such as Crohn's, celiac disease, bacterial overgrowth, or achlorhydria after gastrectomy).
- Gastrointestinal blood loss (e.g., from peptic ulcer disease, esophagitis, occult carcinoma, or angiodysplasia).

History of the patient with anemia

Depending on the severity of anemia and the presence of concurrent pathology, the patient can present with symptoms of anemia such as:

- Fatigue.
- Palpitations.
- Shortness of breath.
- Angina pectoris.

Frequently, the detection of anemia is an incidental finding on a routine blood test when the patient presents with unrelated symptoms.

> Symptoms of anemia such as fatigue are thought to require a reduction in hemoglobin concentration of about 25%. For practical purposes, this means that symptoms are uncommon unless hemoglobin is <8 g/dL (females) or <10 g/dL (males).

The following aspects of the patient history should be considered in detail.

Diet

Check whether the patient has a well-balanced diet:

- Meat contains heme iron, which is more readily bioavailable than nonheme iron.
- Strict vegans are particularly at risk of iron deficiency.
- Fresh vegetables and fruit are important sources of the reductants (e.g., vitamin C) necessary to make iron bioavailable, resulting in the conversion of Fe^{3+} to Fe^{2+}.

Past medical and surgical history

Clearly, previous surgical procedures may be pertinent, such as:

- Partial gastrectomy resulting in achlorhydria and thus preventing reduction of iron.
- Terminal ileal resection, leading to vitamin B_{12} malabsorption.

Previous medical history is important for similar reasons:

- Crohn's disease or tuberculosis can affect terminal ileal absorption.
- Use of nonsteroidal anti-inflammatory agents, including low-dose aspirin, is associated with chronic occult blood loss.

Associated features

Consider the following associated features:

- Diarrhea with anemia is a common manifestation of malabsorption. Chronic diarrhea due to giardiasis or hookworm infestation is a common cause of anemia worldwide. Celiac disease is a common cause of malabsorption presenting with anemia in the Western world.
- Abdominal pain or dyspepsia may be present, suggesting acid reflux or peptic ulcer disease causing chronic gastrointestinal blood loss, although these are not common causes of anemia. Pain may also be present if a luminal tumor is the cause.
- Hematemesis is not usually ignored by patients but melena occasionally is. This may be caused by

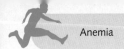

gastric ulcer or erosion, angiodysplasia of the stomach, or a right-sided colonic tumor.

Examining the patient with anemia

Look for features of anemia such as:
- Pallor.
- Koilonychia.
- Atrophic glossitis.
- Tachycardia or cardiac failure.

Check whether there are any abdominal scars from surgery (see Fig. 22.10). The patient may have forgotten about operations, so consider particularly:
- Midline scar of gastric surgery.
- Right lower abdominal or midline scar from an ileal resection.

Can you elicit any abdominal tenderness, and does its position suggest underlying peptic ulcer disease or a cecal carcinoma? (See Fig. 21.1.)

Is there palpable splenomegaly? This may be consequent on portal hypertension or may present as a feature of a myeloproliferative or lymphoproliferative disorder.

Are there features of chronic liver disease, such as spider nevi, parotitis, or gynecomastia, that may alert you to underlying esophageal varices or portal hypertensive gastropathy?

A rectal examination is mandatory in any patient presenting with iron deficiency anemia to exclude anorectal carcinoma. It also serves to confirm or refute a recent history of melena.

Pale conjunctivae correlate very poorly with hemoglobin concentration and cannot be relied on as a sign.

Investigating anemia

The complete blood count is necessary not only to confirm the presence of anemia, but also as an important key to its subsequent investigation. The severity of the anemia is determined by hemoglobin and hematocrit. Important clues to the etiology are often given by the red blood cell size and hemoglobin content. Thus:
- Microcytic hypochromic picture is due to iron deficiency. This can result from dietary deficiency, failure of absorption, or blood loss. A blood film may demonstrate anisocytosis and poikilocytosis (variation in size and shape of the red cell, respectively).
- Normocytic normochromic picture is commonly associated with chronic inflammatory disease, in which iron stores are adequate but not used effectively.
- Macrocytic picture, which can be due to folate or vitamin B_{12} deficiency, alcohol, hypothyroidism, or certain drugs (e.g., phenytoin-antifolate action), or hydroxyurea.

Further investigation, therefore, is dependent on the full blood count indices.

Parameters to differentiate iron-deficiency anemia from anemia of chronic disease		
	Anemia of chronic disease	Iron deficiency
MCV	↓/normal	↓
Serum iron	↓	↓
TIBC	↓	↑
Ferritin	↓/normal/↑	↓
Iron stores in bone marrow (Perls' stain)	normal	↓/absent
Iron in red-cell precursors	↓	↓/absent

Fig. 11.1 Parameters to differentiate iron-deficiency anemia from anemia of chronic disease (MCV, mean corpuscular volume; TIBC, total iron-binding capacity).

Because complete blood counts are automated, macrocytosis can be spurious if increased numbers of larger red cells, such as reticulocytes, are present. If in doubt, a reticulocyte count and a blood film examination should be performed.

- Vitamin B_{12} must also be measured in patients with macrocytosis. If deficient, a Schilling test (see Chapter 24) may be helpful in deciding the cause.
- Blood urea can be a useful, albeit rather unreliable, indicator of nutrition—low levels occur in malabsorption.
- Feces can be tested for occult blood loss, although both false-positive and false-negative results can be obtained.

Biochemistry

Biochemistry tests may aid diagnosis (Fig. 11.1):
- Serum iron is used to confirm iron deficiency.
- Serum ferritin is the most sensitive test to reflect iron stores but, as an "acute-phase protein," its measurement may be falsely elevated in the presence of a concomitant inflammatory condition.
- Serum folate should be measured in any patient with macrocytosis. Deficiency is usually due to malabsorption (most commonly, celiac disease), poor dietary intake, excessive use as in pregnancy, or increased cell turnover in malignancy or red cell hemolysis. Antifolate drugs, such as methotrexate, and antibiotics, such as trimethoprim, also cause folate deficiency.

If macrocytic anemia is due to vitamin B_{12} deficiency because of bacterial overgrowth, serum folate will be elevated as a consequence of bacterial metabolism. Otherwise, folate levels are often also deficient.

Endoscopy

Esophagogastroduodenoscopy should be undertaken in all cases of iron-deficiency anemia, unless there is clearly an alternative explanation, to exclude esophagitis, gastric ulcer or erosions, and carcinoma.

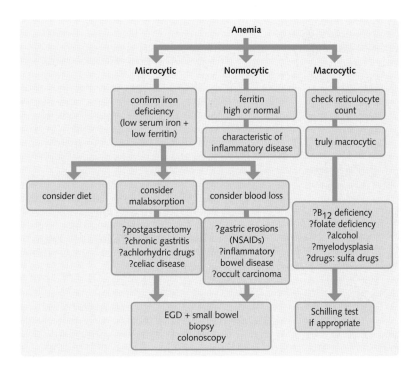

Fig. 11.2 Algorithm for the gastrointestinal investigation of anemia (NSAIDs, nonsteroidal anti-inflammatory drugs; EGD, esophagogastroduodenoscopy).

The presence of a duodenal ulcer is an insufficient explanation for iron-deficiency anemia. A biopsy of the second part of the duodenum should be taken at the same time to exclude celiac disease.

Colonoscopy is the preferred large bowel investigation because it should identify all lesions resulting in blood loss, including angiodysplasia. When it is not practical, barium examination should be undertaken.

Radiology

A barium meal is indicated if there is suspicion of gastric carcinoma and gastroscopy is not possible. Similarly, a barium enema will demonstrate the presence of diverticular disease, polyps, and carcinoma, but endoscopy is preferable to ascribe the cause of bleeding to a particular lesion or to identify angiodysplasia.

Angiography is helpful in the presence of active bleeding but is not generally rewarding in the investigation of chronic anemia.

Other tests for anemia

Other tests may be useful:

- A Schilling test may help differentiate the different causes of vitamin B_{12} deficiency (see Chapter 24).
- A ^{14}C-glycocholic acid breath test or a lactulose hydrogen breath test may be used to investigate bacterial overgrowth (see Chapter 24).
- A ^{99m}Tc radioisotope scan is helpful if a Meckel's diverticulum is suspected of causing chronic anemia in a young patient.
- A ^{51}Cr-labeled red cell scan may give a clue to the general location of occult blood loss, but is not helpful to identify the nature of the lesion or the precise anatomic location.

Summary

An algorithm summarizing the investigation of anemia is given in Fig. 11.2.

12. Jaundice

Jaundice is a yellow coloring of the skin and sclerae due to elevated levels of bilirubin in plasma. Jaundice is usually clinically evident if the serum bilirubin level exceeds 40 mol/L or 3 mg/dL (about twice the normal upper limit). There are numerous causes of jaundice, and a careful history and examination are vital so that unnecessary invasive investigations can be avoided.

The more common causes include:

- Hemolytic anemias or ineffective erythropoiesis such as autoimmune hemolytic anemia or hemoglobinopathies, respectively.
- Congenital hyperbilirubinemia due to enzyme defects—most commonly, Gilbert's syndrome.
- Extrahepatic bile duct obstruction due to gallstones, pancreatitis, or pancreatic cancer.
- Sclerosing cholangitis.
- Intrahepatic cholestasis due to drugs, alcohol, hepatitis, or chronic liver disease.

History of the patient with jaundice

All aspects of the history should be taken with care as there are times when certain facts can appear to be trivial, yet may later become vital in the diagnosis. The following features help to differentiate causes of jaundice (Fig. 12.1).

Age

Younger patients are more likely to have congenital hyperbilirubinemia or viral hepatitis than carcinoma of the pancreas, which rarely affects those aged under 60 years.

Onset of symptoms

The onset of symptoms may give clues to the diagnosis:

- An acute onset is more likely to be of infective or drug-induced etiology.
- A slow insidious onset is more likely to be due to chronic active hepatitis (e.g., caused by autoimmune disease or alcohol).

Infectious contact and risk behavior

It is important to establish whether the patient has any risk factors for developing jaundice.

- Find out whether there has been contact with other people with jaundice, such as occurs in epidemics of hepatitis A and E or infectious mononucleosis (Epstein-Barr virus).
- Has there been high-risk behavior for exposure to hepatitis B (e.g., promiscuous sexual activity or shared needles)?
- A history of recent travel abroad is also essential: ingestion of seafood abroad is a common source of infectious hepatitis. Do not forget exotic causes such as yellow fever contracted while in Africa!
- Occupational or recreational history may be relevant: sewage and farm workers are at risk of leptospirosis, as well as windsurfers and people who go caving/spelunking.
- A history of excess alcohol consumption must be excluded, and tactful discussion with relatives may be necessary.

The most common mode for transmission of hepatitis B worldwide is not sexual or intravenous drugs but "vertical" transmission from mother to baby. This takes place in the birth canal and presents the best opportunity to prevent transmission of hepatitis B virus in the immunization of the neonate.

Past medical history

The patient's past medical history may immediately suggest a diagnosis. For example:

- Previous cholecystectomy could suggest a bile duct stone or stricture.
- Ulcerative colitis can predispose a patient to sclerosing cholangitis.
- Anesthetic agents such as halothane can precipitate jaundice.

Causes of jaundice	
Prehepatic	hemolysis ineffective erythropoesis Gilbert and Crigler-Najjar syndromes

Hepatic	viruses: hepatitis A, B, C, E
	       Epstein-Barr
	       cytomegalovirus
	       herpes simplex/zoster
	
	leptospirosis/toxoplasmosis
	autoimmune hepatitis
	cirrhosis
	Wilson's disease
	rotor/Dubin-Johnson syndrome
	drugs

Posthepatic
(obstructive)
	intrahepatic: primary biliary cirrhosis
	       primary sclerosing cholangitis
	       cholangiocarcinoma
	       drugs
	       + same causes listed under hepatic
	
	extrahepatic: gallstones
	       carcinoma of head of pancreas
	       enlarged lymph nodes at porta hepatis
	       cholangiocarcinoma

Fig. 12.1 Causes of jaundice.

- Patients often forget that they have taken antibiotics or other drugs recently.

Drugs

Many drugs are metabolized in the liver, and some cause idiosyncratic reactions that result in jaundice. Others have a dose-related effect, resulting in liver damage and jaundice. Important drugs to consider include:

- Antibiotics such as amoxicillin/clavulanic acid (Augmentin).
- Antifungal agents such as fluconazole.
- Allopurinol can occasionally cause profound jaundice.
- Antituberculous drugs such as isoniazid or rifampin.
- Neuroleptics such as chlorpromazine.
- Acetaminophen in excess of therapeutic dose.
- Anabolic steroids, which are occasionally illegally used by bodybuilders and cause jaundice.

Family history

A history of intermittent jaundice in the family suggests congenital hyperbilirubinemia. Also, inquire about Wilson's disease and alpha–1-antitrypsin deficiency.

Associated features

A number of features may suggest underlying pathology, such as:

- Presence of abdominal pain. Particularly if localized to right upper quadrant, this suggests bile duct stones or pain originating from the liver capsule.
- Acute onset abdominal distention with jaundice. This may indicate acute hepatitis or hepatic vein thrombosis (resulting in ascites).
- Painless jaundice in conjunction with weight loss in older patients, which is suggestive of carcinoma of the pancreas or enlarged metastatic lymph nodes at the porta hepatis.
- Signs of cardiac failure, especially elevated jugular venous pressure and peripheral edema, which may indicate a congested liver with jaundice.

"Acholuric jaundice" is the term given to jaundice without dark urine and pale stool. The presence of these features indicates that the jaundice is cholestatic in nature. Obstructive jaundice is only one cause of cholestatic jaundice.

Examining the patient with jaundice

Assess the severity of the jaundice clinically:

- Acute jaundice has a bright yellow hue.
- Chronic jaundice has a dusky appearance and, if severe, the patient may look green.

Look for signs of anemia, which may indicate underlying hemolysis or Wilson's disease.

Generalized lymphadenopathy may be due to Epstein-Barr virus infection, cytomegalovirus infection, or toxoplasmosis.

Look for features of chronic liver disease or cirrhosis (see Chapter 18), such as:

- Parotitis.
- Spider nevi.
- Gynecomastia and loss of secondary sexual characteristics.
- Palmar erythema.
- Splenomegaly (think of infections, hemolysis, or portal hypertension).

- Hepatomegaly.
- Ascites (may indicate acute in Budd-Chiari syndrome).

The gallbladder may be palpated in a patient with progressive painless jaundice due to obstruction. If, in painless jaundice, the gallbladder is palpable, the cause will not be gallstones (Courvoisier's law). In elderly patients, this phenomenon is commonly due to carcinoma of the head of the pancreas.

Associated systemic signs may suggest particular syndromes with liver involvement:

- Chronic respiratory disease with jaundice may occur with cystic fibrosis or alpha–1-antitrypsin deficiency.
- Neurologic signs (particularly those of parkinsonism) with jaundice may suggest hepatolenticular degeneration (Wilson's disease).

Kayser-Fleischer rings are present in 70% of patients with Wilson's disease. They are seen as a brown ring around in the periphery of the cornea, most often at the top. Slit-lamp examination may be necessary.

Investigating jaundice

Abdominal ultrasound is the key investigation in a patient with jaundice because it will differentiate obstructive jaundice from other causes, and the subsequent approaches to management are different. If the bile ducts are not dilated, then blood tests become useful to differentiate causes of jaundice:

- Urine testing for bilirubin and urobilinogen is rarely helpful to make a firm diagnosis, but it is inexpensive. Unconjugated jaundice (e.g., Gilbert's syndrome or hemolysis) results in an absence of bilirubin in the urine. Biliary obstruction demonstrates increased urinary bilirubin and absent or reduced urobilinogen. Hemosiderin may be detectable in the presence of active red cell hemolysis.
- Liver biochemistry is helpful to confirm jaundice and to confirm unconjugated hyperbilirubinemia in cases of congenital or hemolytic jaundice. A high

alkaline phosphatase level is indicative of cholestasis, whereas high levels of transaminases are suggestive of a hepatitic cause. However, a mixed picture is often the case; hence, too much emphasis should not be given to blood test results alone.

- Aspartate/alanine aminotransferase greater than 2 is suggestive of alcoholic hepatitis under the right context.
- Prothrombin time is the most easily available test that gives some indication of hepatic synthetic function because all of the clotting factors are made in the liver. It correlates well with outcome in acute liver failure.

Prothrombin time is influenced by vitamin K, which is a required cofactor for coagulation factors II, VII, IX, and X. Because vitamin K is a fat-soluble vitamin, its absorption is reduced in biliary duct obstruction, when sufficient bile fails to reach the small intestine. In this situation, a single dose of intravenous vitamin K may correct the prothrombin time; it will have no effect if the coagulopathy is due to deficient synthesis of coagulation factors, as in parenchymal liver diseases.

- Albumin, also synthesized in the liver, is reduced in any "sick" state and correlates less well with the severity of liver dysfunction. Similarly, blood urea levels are usually low but not very informative.
- The serum bilirubin level does not necessarily reflect the degree of liver damage, particularly in the acute situation. In chronic liver disease, it gives a reasonable indication of the stage of progression.
- Complete blood count may reveal anemia. This may be spuriously macrocytic if accompanied by a significant reticulocytosis, as in hemolytic disease. Reticulocyte count should be checked. Macrocytosis with low platelets is suggestive of hypersplenism associated with the portal hypertension of chronic liver disease. A blood film may be appropriate to look for signs of hemolysis, sickle cells, or atypical lymphocytes seen in Epstein-Barr virus infection (or other viral infections).

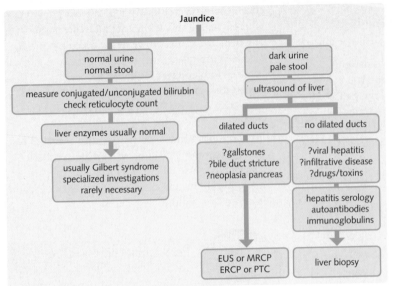

Fig. 12.2 Algorithm for the evaluation of a patient with jaundice (EUS, endoscopic ultrasound; MRCP, magnetic resonance cholangiopancreatography; ERCP, endoscopic retrograde cholangiopancreatography; PTC, percutaneous transhepatic cholangiography).

- Serology should be reserved to look for viral markers of acute hepatitis A to E and for Epstein-Barr virus, cytomegalovirus, and toxoplasmosis. A monospot test can give a rapid diagnosis of infectious mononucleosis. Markers for leptospirosis should also be done if clinically indicated.

- Autoantibodies to nuclear proteins and smooth muscle indicate an acute autoimmune hepatitis. They will usually be accompanied by elevated immunoglobulin (Ig) G levels. IgA is commonly elevated in alcoholic hepatitis. IgM (specifically, the M_2 subtype) is elevated in primary biliary cirrhosis.

- Elevated urinary copper and low serum ceruloplasmin levels indicate the possibility of Wilson's disease, which is fatal if undetected and untreated.

- Percutaneous liver biopsy can provide valuable information regarding both the cause and extent of parenchymal liver damage. It is usually performed under ultrasound guidance, and the prothrombin time must be checked before biopsy. Special staining for copper and alpha–1-antitrypsin can be performed on histologic sections.

- A computed tomography scan of the abdomen is mainly used to assess pancreatic masses and nodes at the porta hepatis when obstructive jaundice has been confirmed by ultrasound.

- Magnetic resonance cholangiography and endoscopic ultrasound are useful examinations for assessment of the bile duct, while obviating the serious risk of acute pancreatitis associated with an endoscopic retrograde cholangiopancreatography (ERCP).

- ERCP or percutaneous transhepatic cholangiography is useful for further assessment and therapy if obstruction is identified.

Summary

An algorithm summarizing the investigation of a patient with jaundice is shown in Fig. 12.2.

DISEASES AND DISORDERS

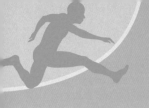

Anatomy, physiology, and function of the esophagus

The esophagus is a muscular tube composed of two layers:

- An outer longitudinal layer.
- An inner circular muscle layer.

The esophagus connects the pharynx to the stomach. Striated (voluntary) muscle in the upper portion gradually changes to smooth muscle in the lower part and then becomes continuous with the muscle layer of the stomach. The lining of the esophagus also changes from a stratified squamous epithelium to columnar epithelium at the gastroesophageal junction (Fig. 14.1).

When a food bolus is propelled into the pharynx by the tongue, the upper esophageal sphincter (controlled by cricopharyngeus muscle) relaxes, allowing the passage of food into the esophagus. A primary peristaltic wave starts from the pharynx and continues down along the length of the esophagus. Secondary peristalsis occurs locally due to distention of the esophagus by a food bolus. The lower esophageal sphincter (LES) relaxes prior to peristaltic contractions when swallowing is initiated. The progression of a peristaltic swallow wave can be followed by placing

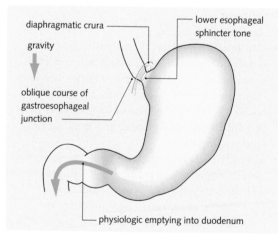

Fig. 14.1 Anatomic relations of the esophagus.

pressure transducers at intervals along the esophagus (esophageal manometry; see Figs. 24.9 and 24.10).

Preventing regurgitation of the stomach contents back into the esophagus is dependent on:

- Gravity.
- LES pressure.
- The oblique course of the gastroesophageal junction.
- The diaphragmatic crura wrapped around the esophagus.
- The physiologic emptying of the stomach contents into the duodenum through the pylorus.

Inflammatory conditions

Reflux esophagitis
Incidence
The incidence of reflux esophagitis, a common condition, increases with age. The cause is probably multifactorial but may be related to the fact that hiatal hernias are found more commonly in elderly persons.

Clinical features
Various symptoms are associated with the reflux of gastric acid contents into the esophagus. When the symptoms produce upper abdominal pain, belching, or heartburn, they are referred to collectively as "dyspepsia" (see Chapter 1). Otherwise, more specific terms should be used to describe them:

- Heartburn is the most common presenting symptom due to reflux of gastric acid into the esophagus. This can cause erosive esophagitis. Correlation between symptoms and extent of esophagitis is poor.
- Retrosternal chest pain can be due to spasm of the distal esophageal muscle or inflammation.
- Vomiting of blood (i.e., hematemesis) can occur in association with severe esophagitis.
- Iron-deficiency anemia can occur due to insidious blood loss from chronic inflammation.

- Nocturnal cough and early morning bronchospasm, producing a dip in peak flow readings, may occur as a result of reflux with microaspiration into the trachea. There is some evidence that acid in the esophagus can precipitate reflex bronchospasm (see Fig. 1.1).

Do not forget to consider medication as a cause or precipitant for dyspepsic/reflux-type symptoms. Many drugs can be implicated—especially those with anticholinergic effects. If in doubt, check!

Diagnosis and investigation
Endoscopy
Endoscopy may reveal the varying grades of esophagitis and, in severe cases, ulceration. However, normal endoscopy does not exclude reflux esophagitis, and a biopsy may be necessary.

Twenty-four hour intraluminal pH monitoring
Twenty-four hour intraluminal pH monitoring is probably the most accurate way of detecting reflux disease because there is a reasonable correlation between low pH (4) occurring within the 24-hour period and symptoms of reflux (see Figs. 24.11 and 24.12). Manometry should be done if surgery is considered in patients with esophagitis refractory to medical treatment.

Cine esophagogram
Cine esophagography is still used but its results are significant only when a free reflux of barium is demonstrated.

Etiology and pathogenesis
A reduction in tone of the LES is the main factor contributing to acid reflux. This normally occurs when the patient lies down or if there is raised intra-abdominal pressure (e.g., pregnancy, obesity, weight lifting, chronic constipation). Reduction in the resistance of the esophageal mucosa to acid and delayed gastric emptying will also predispose the patient to acid reflux. Any drug with an anticholinergic action (e.g., tricyclic antidepressants, antipsychotics, oxybutynin, theophylline) may aggravate symptoms of reflux. Nonsteroidal anti-inflammatory drugs can also contribute to symptoms.

Alcohol consumption and smoking have also been implicated in its pathogenesis: smoking reduces LES tone, and alcohol stimulates gastric acid production.

A sliding-type hiatal hernia, in which the gastroesophageal junction lies above the diaphragm, is associated with esophageal reflux. However, its presence alone is not diagnostic because not all patients with hiatal hernia will develop symptoms.

Complications
Stricture
Stricture occurs after long-standing acid reflux, causing stricture of the lower esophagus and producing symptoms of dysphagia.

Barrett's esophagus
Replacement of squamous cells with columnar cells may occur with chronic reflux. Cells that develop other abnormal features may become dysplastic with potential for malignant transformation. This may be prevented or possibly even reversed by antireflux therapy.

Prognosis
More than 50% of patients will have significant improvement with only conservative treatment.

Aims of treatment
Treatment is undertaken mainly for symptom control. Barrett's esophagus should be treated, and surveillance for development of dysplastic features should be undertaken by endoscopy.

Treatment
Treatment may include:
- Conservative treatments, such as weight reduction, cessation of smoking, and reduction in alcohol consumption. These courses will help symptoms in mild cases. If reflux is mainly nocturnal, raising the head of the bed may be of benefit. Eating regular meals and avoiding fatty food are important.
- Antacids, such as magnesium trisilicate or alginate-containing compounds. These coat the mucosa and will abolish symptoms in most mild cases.
- H_2-receptor antagonists (e.g., nizatidine or ranitidine), which work by reducing gastric acid output as a result of histamine H_2-receptor blockade.

- Proton pump inhibitors (e.g., omeprazole or lansoprazole), which are potent inhibitors of acid production. This is achieved by blocking the hydrogen-potassium adenosine triphosphate enzyme system (the "proton-pump") of the gastric parietal cell. It is the drug class of choice for severe symptoms and Barrett's esophagus because there is almost complete inhibition of acid production from the stomach.
- Prokinetic drugs (e.g., domperidone), which can enhance gut motility, probably by increasing the release of dopamine or acetylcholine. (Cisapride was a similar drug that improved gastric emptying and concomitantly increased LES pressure but has now been withdrawn because it predisposed patients to dangerous cardiac arrhythmias.)
- Surgery. Tightening the lower esophagus by wrapping the fundus of the stomach around it (fundoplication) is reserved for patients who are symptomatic despite compliance with conservative and pharmacologic treatment. This procedure can be performed safely and successfully via laparoscopy, but patients should be carefully selected. Too tight a wrap results in dysphagia.

Barrett's esophagus
Incidence
About 15% of patients with prolonged reflux of acid into the lower esophagus have Barrett's esophagus.

Etiology and pathogenesis
Prolonged irritation causes the transformation (metaplasia) from squamous epithelium to columnar-type intestinal epithelium, which is covered by mucin (Fig. 14.2). Intestinal metaplastic change is occasionally followed by dysplastic change predisposing to malignant transformation.

Clinical features
The clinical features of Barrett's esophagus are the same as those of reflux esophagitis.

Diagnosis and investigation
Seen at endoscopy, where normal squamous epithelium is replaced by columnar epithelium (metaplasia). Barrett's esophagus manifests endoscopically as a change of texture and of color from pink to slightly orange. Chromoendoscopy is currently being evaluated for diagnosis of dysplasia in Barrett's esophagus. Histologic examination will confirm the diagnosis, revealing varying grades of cellular change from metaplasia through to severe dysplasia.

Complications
Barrett's esophagus predisposes to adenocarcinoma of the esophagus. This tumor has an increasing prevalence throughout the developed world. It is thought to carry up to a 40-fold risk of adenocarcinoma. Absence of the tumor suppressor gene p53 may have etiologic relevance.

Prognosis
Prognosis depends on grade of dysplasia, cessation of reflux, and endoscopic surveillance. Adequate treatment with a proton pump inhibitor abolishes symptoms of reflux and may allow columnar epithelium to return to normal squamous epithelium, thus avoiding premalignant change.

Treatment
Proton pump inhibitors such as omeprazole may be given long term to prevent recurrence. Repeated endoscopies may be required to monitor dysplastic change, if present. Techniques such as epithelial laser ablation or photodynamic therapy intend to result in resolution of metaplasia, but the long-term outcome is not known.

Esophageal strictures
Incidence
Benign strictures secondary to acid reflux are becoming less common among those with gastroesophageal reflux disease because of the availability of H_2 antagonists and proton pump inhibitors.

Clinical features
Dysphagia, or difficulty in swallowing, is the main presenting symptom of esophageal stricture. This can be progressive from solids to liquids as fibrosis worsens.

Weight loss can be marked because the patient may have difficulty maintaining the required caloric intake. The patient may often give a history of preceding reflux that disappeared before the onset of dysphagia. This happens because the development of a fibrotic stricture can impair further reflux of acid. Symptoms can mimic malignant stricture, although benign strictures tend to have a longer symptomatic history.

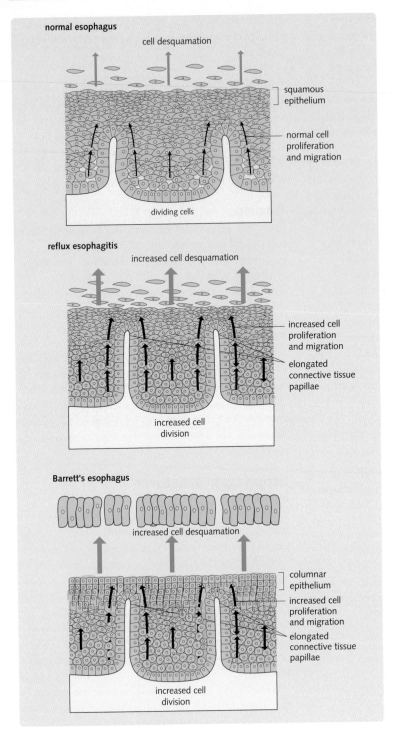

Fig. 14.2 Changes in Barrett's mucosa: the normal squamous epithelium is replaced by columnar epithelium. Cells with abnormal nuclear material constitute dysplastic change and herald malignant transformation.

Diagnosis and investigation

Consider the following investigations:

- Endoscopy can show extensive scarring of the esophagus, and biopsy is necessary to exclude malignant disease.

- Barium swallow or cine esophagogram is an alternative if the patient cannot tolerate endoscopy. A smooth diffuse stricture can be seen usually without shouldering.

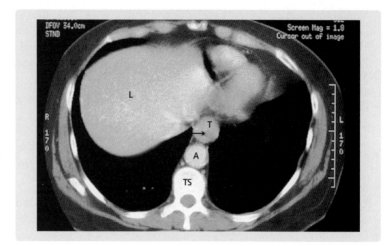

Fig. 14.3 Computed tomography scan demonstrating malignant infiltration from an esophageal stricture. Only a pinhole lumen remains of the esophagus (arrow), which is surrounded by tumor (T) (A, aorta; L, liver; TS, thoracic spine).

- Imaging by endoluminal ultrasound or a spiral computed tomography scan may be necessary to exclude malignant infiltration (Fig. 14.3).

Etiology and pathogenesis
Long-standing acid reflux causes permanent scarring and fibrosis. Other causes include:
- Ingestion of caustic substance.
- Previous radiotherapy.
- Previous sclerotherapy for esophageal varices.
- Prolonged intubation of a nasogastric tube.

Complications
There is an increased incidence of malignant change in benign strictures, but this may reflect the underlying pathology.

Prognosis
Once a stricture has formed, the condition is likely to remain throughout life.

Aim of treatment
The aim of treatment is purely for symptomatic relief of dysphagia. Reflux should also be treated to prevent worsening of the condition.

Treatment
Treatment may include the following:
- Dilatation is undertaken endoscopically with graduated tubes of increasing sizes inserted through the affected part of the esophagus to widen the lumen. The procedure often needs to be repeated because renarrowing of the lumen can

occur over time. Endoscopic balloon dilatation is an alternative that is probably safer. Esophageal perforation is a small but significant procedure-related risk.
- Surgery is required if dilatation fails to control symptoms of dysphagia.

Neoplasia

Carcinoma of the esophagus
Incidence
Carcinoma of the esophagus occurs in approximately 10,000 persons in the United States. A higher rate is seen in parts of China and Africa, possibly related to local diet.

Clinical features
Dysphagia is the most common presenting symptom and is progressive from solids to liquids. This can occur relatively rapidly over a period of weeks to months.
Other features include:
- Weight loss—consequent upon anorexia and dysphagia, and possibly mediated by the release of tumor cytokines.
- Anemia due to ulceration of the lesion, which is common and may cause insidious blood loss, resulting in iron-deficiency anemia.
- Pain on swallowing (odynophagia). This occurs in advanced stages; local infiltration by the tumor causes diffuse, persistent, retrosternal pain.
- Dyspnea and cough, due to aspiration of pharyngeal secretions. In advanced cases, this may

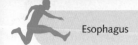

be due to esophagotracheal fistulas or tracheal encasement.

Diagnosis and investigation

Consider the following investigations:

- Complete blood count may demonstrate iron-deficiency anemia or pancytopenia from metastatic bone marrow infiltration by tumor.
- Derangement of liver biochemistry or hypercalcemia may be seen if metastases are present.
- Urea and electrolyte levels often reveal dehydration, as a result of dysphagia.
- Endoscopy is the investigation of choice because it allows direct visualization of the lesion and an opportunity for biopsy and histologic confirmation.
- Barium swallow is reserved for patients who cannot tolerate an endoscopy or those suspected of having a high-level stricture. Malignant strictures characteristically have a shouldered appearance (see Fig. 2.3, B).
- Endoscopic ultrasound and spiral computed tomography scan of the thorax are used for staging if surgery is under consideration. Commonly, this is precluded by the frailty of the patient, late presentation with advanced malignancy, or concomitant medical conditions.

Etiology and pathogenesis

Carcinoma of the esophagus rarely occurs in patients younger than 50 years of age. Two histologic types are seen:

- Squamous carcinoma.
- Adenocarcinoma.

Squamous carcinoma

- Ninety percent of all esophageal cancer is squamous in nature, but adenocarcinoma is increasing in the United States and other Western countries.
- Fifty percent of all squamous cancers occur in the lower third of esophagus.
- There is a higher incidence in China, which may suggest a dietary etiology.
- This type of carcinoma is more common in men, particularly those with a high alcohol intake and a history of cigarette smoking.

- The more unusual predisposing factors include achalasia, Plummer-Vinson syndrome, and tylosis (i.e., hyperkeratosis of palms and soles inherited as a rare autosomal dominant condition).

Adenocarcinoma

- Usually as a result of malignant transformation of Barrett's esophagus.
- Occasionally, arises as an extension from adenocarcinoma of gastric cardia.

Complications

The tumor may invade adjacent anatomic structures:

- Through the esophageal wall and into a bronchus, creating an esophageal-bronchial fistula, resulting in recurrent pneumonia (note that aspiration pneumonia may occur as a result of severe dysphagia, in the absence of a fistula).
- Into the thoracic aorta, resulting in rapid exsanguination.

Prognosis

To some extent, prognosis is dependent on the stage of the tumor and the fitness of the patient. However, the prognosis is usually exceptionally poor, with an overall survival of 2% at 5 years.

Treatment

Treatment is mainly palliative because curative treatment is rarely possible due to late presentation of the disease. Consider the following options:

- Surgery provides the only possible cure but carries an operative mortality rate of 5–10%. Less than 40% of patients are suitable for surgical resection at presentation, but these patients are often elderly and frail with medical comorbidity precluding radical surgery.
- Radiotherapy reduces the bulk of the tumor and may relieve dysphagia. Fistula formation is more common after radiotherapy treatment.
- High-energy thermal laser ablation is used to burn through the bulk of the tumor and restore the esophageal lumen. An alternative for smaller tumors is photodynamic therapy, using a lower-energy laser light in combination with a chemical photosensitizer, which is selectively taken up by tumor tissue. Repeated administration of either modality may be required.

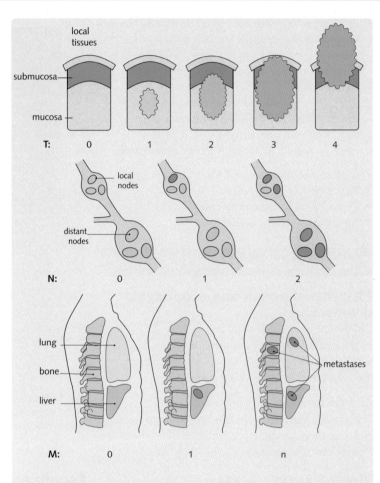

Fig. 14.4 Graphic illustration of the tumor-node-metastasis (TNM) classification of mucosal malignant disease. T0, no evidence of primary tumor; T1, tumor confined to mucosa; T2, infiltration through submucosa but not penetrating through the muscularis; T3, extends through muscularis to serosa; T4, extends to surrounding tissues; N0, no lymph node involvement; N1, local lymph node involvement; N2, distant lymph node involvement; M0, no metastasis; M1, metastasis.

T = graded 0–4; refers to the primary tumor according to its depth of involvement
T0 = no evidence of primary tumor

N = 0–2; refers to lymph nodes involved; increasing score indicates higher numbers of lymph node involvement

M = 0 or 1; refers to presence or absence of metastasis. The example shown might be for carcinoma of the colon

- Endoscopic placement of a plastic or expanding metal hollow stent (endoprosthesis) across the obstructing lesion can give palliative relief of dysphagia. This carries a risk of perforation in up to 10% of patients.

Tumor-node-metastasis classification of tumors

The approach to management of many malignant tumors depends on their stage. In addition, a comparison of treatment strategies is heavily reliant on making sure that like is compared with like.

An internationally accepted classification for tumors is the tumor-node-metastasis (TNM) staging system. This system varies for different organs and tissues but follows the general principle shown in Fig. 14.4.

- "T" refers to the extent of the tumor itself: T0 usually indicates no detectable tumor, T1 indicates the tumor is confined to the mucosa, T3 indicates infiltration of deeper layers or surrounding structures, depending on the site, and T4 indicates extension beyond the serosa and invasion of surrounding tissues.

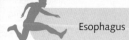

- "N" refers to lymph node involvement: N0 means no node involvement, N1 usually indicates that the tumor is confined to local nodes, and N2 means confined to more distant nodes specified for that tumor type.
- Very distant nodes are usually classified as "M" for metastatic: M0 means no metastasis detected, and "Mn" indicates distant spread, with "n" having a specific meaning for each tumor type.

Thus, a tumor classified as T4N2M2 is one with:
- Extensive local infiltration.
- Distant lymph node involvement.
- Metastatic spread to other sites.

Anatomic and functional problems

Pharyngeal pouch and esophageal diverticulum

Incidence
Pharyngeal pouch and esophageal diverticulum are usually discovered coincidentally when a barium meal is performed for other reasons.

Clinical features
The majority of these problems are asymptomatic, although they can cause regurgitation of food and are a rare cause of dysphagia.

Diagnosis and investigation
Barium swallow demonstrates the size and location of the lesion (Fig. 14.5).

Etiology and pathogenesis
The cause is probably related to dysmotility of cricopharyngeus muscle and inferior constrictor forming a mucosal outpouching (pharyngeal pouch). Diverticula may also occur in the mid esophagus due to traction by mediastinal lymph node inflammation (traction diverticulum) or just above the LES (epiphrenic diverticulum).

Complications
Complications occur rarely. Perforation may occur when endoscopy is performed for investigation of dysphagia because the pouch may be mistaken for the esophageal lumen!

Treatment
Surgical resection is reserved for pouches that are problematic.

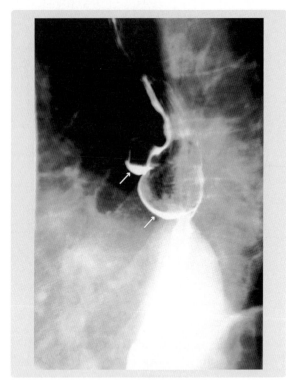

Fig. 14.5 Lateral view of esophageal diverticulum (arrows) in the upper esophagus seen on barium swallow. Note the fluid levels.

Esophageal webs

Incidence
Esophageal web is often a coincidental finding on barium meal. Those associated with iron-deficiency anemia are rare.

Clinical features
Usually the patient is asymptomatic, but high-level dysphagia may occur when tough fibrous food is swallowed without care. There may be a history of a persistent cough due to the aspiration of pharyngeal secretions.

Anemia may present as part of the Plummer-Vinson syndrome (see below).

Diagnosis and investigation
- Barium swallow—demonstrates narrowing of the esophagus by fibrous tissue. The proximal part of the esophagus may be distended with barium.
- Endoscopy—webs may be difficult to see, especially those in the postcricoid area.

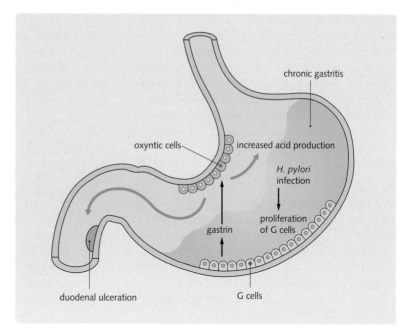

Fig. 15.3 Pathophysiologic representation of mechanisms of *H. pylori*–induced gastritis.

Prognosis and treatment

Patients usually recover without any long-term complications. The removal of the offending cause is usually all that is required. An acute GI bleed should be treated in the conventional way. An H_2 antagonist may be of help in some cases.

Peptic ulcer disease

Under the heading of peptic ulcer disease, we include gastritis, gastric ulcer, and duodenal ulcer, which are dealt with here rather than in Chapter 16. These conditions are all associated with *H. pylori* infection.

Helicobacter pylori infection
Incidence

It is estimated that, in developed countries, 50% of the population over the age of 50 years is infected with the spiral-shaped gram-negative *H. pylori* bacterium. The incidence is declining with improved sanitation, and there is evidence that infection is most often acquired in childhood. In certain parts of the world (e.g., South America), the majority of the population is infected.

Clinical features

Asymptomatic infection is often discovered incidentally. Furthermore, the high prevalence of *H. pylori* infection in certain populations (e.g., Nigeria), without a concomitant, active disease process such as duodenal ulceration, indicates that host factors also have a role in producing pathology and symptoms.

Symptoms suggestive of acute gastritis, chronic gastritis, or peptic ulcer disease usually unmask the presence of *H. pylori* (Fig. 15.3).

Epidemiologic data suggest that there is an increased risk of gastric carcinoma, and long-standing gastritis increases the risk of gastric lymphoma.

Diagnosis and evaluation
The following tests may be useful:

- Endoscopy may demonstrate a blotchy mucosal appearance, and a biopsy specimen can be taken for urease test, histology, or culture to confirm the presence of *H. pylori*.
- In a urease test, an antral biopsy is added to a preprepared urea solution containing a color reagent. If bacterial urease is present, ammonia is produced and reacts with the reagent to produce a color change that is indicative of the presence of the bacterium.
- The bacteria can be detected histologically by routine section and staining.
- A culture can be achieved in special medium.
- With a urea breath test, ^{14}C- or ^{13}C-radiolabeled urea is given orally and *H. pylori* will break it down to ammonia and radiolabeled CO_2, which is

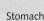

absorbed and subsequently measured in the exhaled breath (see Fig. 24.8).

- In serology, a relatively specific antibody (immunoglobulin G class) can now be measured in serum using an enzyme-linked immunosorbent assay technique, but its clinical value is limited because it confirms past exposure rather than current infection and is not helpful in confirming eradication.
- Stool can also be examined for *H. pylori* antigen.

Etiology and pathogenesis

The exact mechanism remains obscure, but it is thought that persons infected with *H. pylori* have an elevated level of gastrin due to G-cell hyperplasia in the antrum, which, in turn, predisposes the patients to gastric and duodenal ulceration. There may also be an increase in parietal cell mass and pepsinogen production.

Normal gastric mucosa concentrates vitamin C, and its secretion is suppressed by *H. pylori*. This may account for the increased incidence of gastric lymphoma and carcinoma that can occur due to loss of antioxidant activity mediated by ascorbic acid.

Most persons are infected during childhood and have been associated with overcrowded living conditions. The incidence of infection in many countries is falling as a result of improved living conditions.

Complications

Complication of *H. pylori* infection include:
- Acute GI bleed, due to peptic ulcer disease.
- Gastric lymphoma of a particular variety, known as "maltoma" or "MALT lymphoma," has been associated with *Helicobacter* infection. This is a proliferative disease of the mucosa-associated lymphoid tissue (MALT). Reports of regression after *H. pylori* eradication therapy have been published.

Prognosis

Complete eradication is possible for most patients, and the reinfection rate is low.

Treatment

Different treatment regimens have been described. The most successful regimens currently used involve triple therapy with two antibiotics and acid inhibition with a proton pump inhibitor (PPI). The antibiotics used are a combination of amoxicillin, clarithromycin, and metronidazole. Currently, this type of triple-therapy regimen, administered as a twice-daily dose for 7 days, achieves eradication in approximately 90% of patients. (See text under Treatment for Gastric ulcer and Duodenal ulcer.)

 Any patient receiving metronidazole must avoid consuming alcohol because the drug can inhibit acetaldehyde dehydrogenase and produce unpleasant histamine-induced symptoms if this metabolite builds up. This can manifest as facial flushing, headache, palpitations, vomiting, and even cardiac arrhythmias.

Chronic gastritis
Incidence

Current knowledge regarding chronic gastritis includes the following:
- Chronic gastritis can be a progression of acute gastritis.
- *H. pylori* gastritis is by far the most common etiologic factor.
- Autoimmune gastritis is associated with other autoimmune diseases.

Clinical features

Clinical features of chronic gastritis include the following:
- Most cases are asymptomatic.
- Symptoms are similar to those of acute gastritis but occur over a period of time.
- Pernicious anemia due to loss of intrinsic factor secretion for vitamin B_{12} absorption occurs in patients with autoimmune gastritis.

Diagnosis and evaluation

Endoscopy reveals an atrophic mucosa. Intrinsic factor autoantibodies and antiparietal cell antibodies are positive in patients with pernicious anemia.

Etiology and pathogenesis

H. pylori is the most common cause of chronic gastritis. Chronic ingestion of alcohol and NSAIDs may also be contributory, and reflux of bile has also been implicated.

There is loss of parietal and chief cells together with an infiltration of the lamina propria with plasma cells and lymphocytes. Chronic atrophic changes cause intestinal metaplasia.

Autoantibodies to parietal cells and intrinsic factor cause achlorhydria and pernicious anemia, with atrophic changes seen in the stomach.

Complications

Intestinal metaplasia predisposes a patient to malignancy.

Treatment

The aim is to treat the underlying cause:
- Eradication therapy is given for *H. pylori*.
- Vitamin B_{12} is given intramuscularly if pernicious anemia is present.

Gastric ulcer
Incidence

More commonly seen in the elderly population, gastric ulceration is less common than duodenal ulceration by a ratio of 1:4. Peak incidence occurs between the ages of 50 and 60 years.

Clinical features

Epigastric pain can be the main presenting feature. Classically, pain with gastric ulcer is associated with food, whereas duodenal ulcers tend to cause symptoms at night or with an empty stomach and are relieved by food. However, in the majority of cases, the discriminating value of these histories is poor and not helpful in the diagnosis.

Temporary relief with antacids is usually reported.

Associated features include nausea, heartburn, anorexia, and weight loss. These symptoms also occur with gastric carcinoma.

 Be aware that patients often have no pain as a result of gastric ulceration, particularly those cases associated with NSAIDs. They may present with a "painless" acute GI bleed.

Diagnosis and evaluation

Relevant tests for gastric ulcer include:
- Endoscopy, the investigation of choice because biopsy enables differentiation of benign from malignant ulcers. In the case of an acute bleed

from a vessel, an injection of adrenaline may halt the bleeding.
- Barium meal. This will also demonstrate gastric and duodenal ulceration, but biopsies cannot be performed to exclude underlying malignancy.

Etiology and pathogenesis

The exact etiology is unknown, but *H. pylori* infection is present in 70% of cases of gastric ulcer, and most of the remainder are associated with NSAIDs. Some patients with gastric ulcers have normal or low acid output, especially ulcers occurring at the lesser curve of the stomach. Theories regarding pathogenesis include:
- A possible defect in the mucosal barrier, usually maintained by bicarbonate secretion by the gastric epithelium.
- Deficient prostaglandin-mediated cytoprotection. This may account for the higher incidence seen in elderly persons because this cytoprotective mechanism diminishes with age.

Prepyloric ulcers are associated with a high acid output and behave more like a duodenal ulcer.

Differences between malignant and benign gastric ulcers are shown in Fig. 15.4.

Complications

Iron-deficiency anemia is common. Acute GI bleed, perforation, or erosion can occur. Prepyloric ulcers may cause pyloric stenosis and resultant gastric outlet

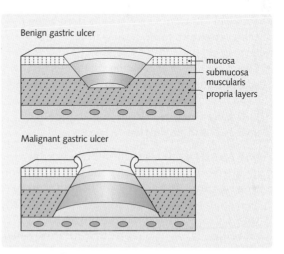

Fig. 15.4 Differences between malignant and benign gastric ulcers. Usually benign ulcers are more superficial. Malignant ulcers have more heaped edges. Multiple biopsy is essential.

obstruction, but this is more commonly seen with duodenal ulcers.

Prognosis

Fifty percent of gastric ulcers recur within 1 year. It has been suggested that long-term antisecretory medication with H_2-receptor antagonists or PPIs should be used.

Treatment

For *H. pylori*–positive ulcers, a triple-therapy eradication regimen with acid suppression is used. There is no known single best eradication regimen, but the following regimens are recommended:

- First-line treatment of 1-week duration consists of PPI (standard dose twice daily) plus amoxicillin (1 g twice daily) or metronidazole (400 mg twice daily), plus clarithromycin (500 mg twice daily). It is sensible to avoid metronidazole if the patient has had a previous course of treatment with this agent.
- Second-line, quadruple therapy consists of PPI (standard dose twice daily), bismuth subcitrate (poorly tolerated), metronidazole (three times daily), and tetracycline four times daily.

Compliance with treatment has been shown to be very important in determining the success of triple-therapy regimens. The eradication course should be followed by antisecretory therapy for 2 months because gastric ulcers tend to take longer to heal than duodenal ulcers.

H. pylori–negative ulcers should be treated with standard antisecretory therapy for 2 months with cessation of NSAIDs where possible (see below).

Other strategies to aid healing include the following:

- Sucralfate, which acts by mucosal protection against action of pepsin, can be useful in resistant cases.
- Discourage smoking because it is linked to increased acid production.

Where NSAID use is clinically desirable, certain strategies can be used to reduce the risk of further mucosal damage:

- Misoprostol is a synthetic prostaglandin analog with antisecretory and mucosa-protective properties. It can help prevent NSAID-associated ulcers.
- Concomitant use of a PPI with NSAIDs is sometimes used in clinical practice, although this strategy is recommended only for patients with a documented NSAID-induced ulcer who must unavoidably continue with NSAID therapy (e.g., severe rheumatoid arthritis).
- Cyclo-oxygenase 2 selective (COX–2) inhibitors (e.g., celecoxib) have a lower incidence of adverse upper GI effects. However, they should be reserved for specific indications (e.g., patients with a history of peptic ulceration, those who are 65 years or older, or those taking concomitant medications predisposing to peptic ulceration).
- There is no evidence to justify the combination of PPIs and COX–2 inhibitors as an additional strategy to prevent adverse gastric effects.

Surgical treatment, such as partial gastrectomy and vagotomy, is reserved for complications of ulceration such as perforation or uncontrolled bleeding.

 Repeat endoscopy with biopsies is essential until a gastric ulcer has completely healed because of the small risk of neoplasia. If the ulcer remains unhealed for 6 months, surgery should be considered.

Duodenal ulcer

Incidence

Approximately 15% of the population will have suffered from duodenal ulceration at some time.

Clinical features

The history of a patient with duodenal ulcer is one of predominantly epigastric pain, often intermittent. Classically, duodenal ulcers are said to be relieved by food or antacids and made worse by hunger. Patients can sometimes point to a specific site of pain in the epigastrium. They can also present with an acute GI bleed.

Diagnosis and evaluation

Diagnosis and evaluation are the same as for gastric ulceration (i.e., endoscopy and biopsy). Tests for *H. pylori* infection should also be performed.

Etiology and pathogenesis

Etiology and pathogenesis of duodenal ulcer are similar to that described for gastric ulceration (i.e., acid production, reduction in cytoprotection). The relationship between *H. pylori* infection and duodenal ulcers is more closely linked because 95% of patients with duodenal ulcers are infected with *H. pylori*. The exact pathogenic mechanism remains uncertain.

High acid output states are associated with duodenal ulceration, as seen in Zollinger-Ellison syndrome. However, more than two thirds of patients have acid secretion within normal limits, which suggests that other factors, such as mucosal barrier and prostaglandin cytoprotection, are involved in its pathogenesis.

Environmental factors such as smoking and psychological stress are associated with increased basal output of acid and NSAIDs reduce prostaglandin production, hence predisposing to ulceration.

First-degree relatives are at three times the normal risk of developing duodenal ulceration. Blood group O has a 40% increase in risk compared with the general population, especially those who do not secrete group O–related antigen in their gastric mucous glycoprotein.

Complications

Complications associated with duodenal ulcer include acute GI bleed, especially if there is an erosion of an artery. Perforation can present as an acute abdominal emergency, and gastric outlet obstruction can occur with chronic disease.

Prognosis

Duodenal ulcer is typically a recurrent disease, and approximately 80% of patients relapse within 1 year if no maintenance or eradication therapy is given. Follow-up is not usually necessary in asymptomatic patients.

Treatment

The strategies taken in treating duodenal ulcer are similar to those for gastric ulceration.

Confirmation of *H. pylori* infection is preferable before an eradication scheme is begun. However, some authorities advocate that eradication therapy should be given to all patients with duodenal ulceration because the correlation with *H. pylori* infection is so high.

Iron-deficiency (hypochromic microcytic) anemia due to chronic blood loss is unusual in duodenal ulcers. If it is present, coexisting pathology must be sought, such as carcinoma of the colon.

Neoplasia of the stomach

Gastric polyps

Incidence

Incidence of gastric polyps is rare. They are discovered, often coincidentally, during approximately 2% of endoscopies.

Clinical features

The majority of cases of gastric polyps are asymptomatic. Occasionally, they may ulcerate and bleed.

Diagnosis and evaluation

Investigations that may be of use include:
- Endoscopy for dyspepsia or abdominal pain, which often identifies polyps incidentally. If multiple polyps are present, then conditions such as Peutz-Jeghers syndrome and familial polyposis coli should be considered. The latter has particular significance because of its malignant potential.
- Biopsy for histologic examination, which will usually confirm the nature of the polyp.
- Endoscopic ultrasound, which may be necessary to exclude submucosal malignant infiltration.

Etiology and pathogenesis

- Over 90% of polyps are hyperplastic, and they are usually nonsinister.
- Approximately 5% of polyps are adenomas and have similar premalignant potential as those found in the colon.

Rarely, patients with pernicious anemia have polyps in the fundus, which may subsequently turn out to be carcinoid tumors. These may be due to the trophic effects of gastrin secondary to achlorhydria.

Complications

Bleeding and malignant change are the usual complications.

Prognosis and treatment

Resection of the polyps will abolish the malignant risk. They can be removed endoscopically via a snare, but those that are large or sessile may not be suitable for this manner of treatment; hence, multiple biopsy specimens are usually taken, and local surgical resection may be required. Hyperplastic polyps are usually left alone unless the patient is symptomatic (Fig. 15.5).

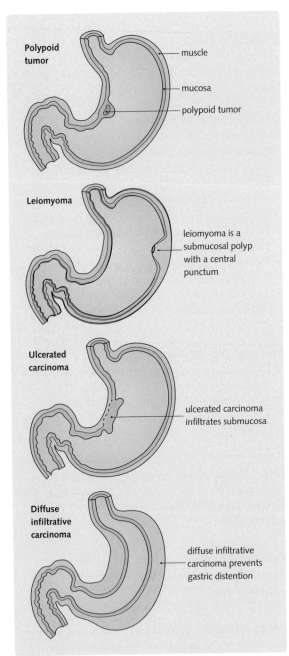

Fig. 15.5 Types of gastric polyps and contrast with leiomyoma and carcinoma.

Gastric leiomyoma

Incidence
Gastric leiomyoma is the most common tumor of the stomach. Autopsy studies have shown the tumor to be present in up to 50% of the population over the age of 50 years.

Clinical features
Small tumors are asymptomatic. Larger tumors may ulcerate or bleed, causing abdominal pain that can be mistaken for peptic ulcer disease.

Diagnosis and evaluation
A leiomyoma is often identified incidentally during an endoscopy carried out for other reasons such as epigastric pain or anemia.

Etiology and pathogenesis
Gastric leiomyoma is a benign tumor of the smooth muscle cells, which are submucosal and covered by intact mucosa. Underlying etiology is unknown.

Treatment
Local resection is curative.

Leiomyosarcoma

Incidence
Leiomyosarcoma accounts for 1% of gastric malignancy.

Clinical features
Clinical features of leiomyosarcoma are similar to those of leiomyoma, except weight loss can be a marked feature. A palpable mass in the epigastrium can be demonstrated in approximately 50% of cases. Larger tumors are more likely to have metastasized at the time of diagnosis to local lymph nodes and lungs.

Treatment
Surgical resection is the treatment of choice.

Ménétrier's disease

Incidence
Ménétrier's disease occurs rarely.

Clinical features
Clinical features include:
- Abdominal pain, vomiting, or bleeding similar to that which occurs in chronic gastritis.
- Hypoalbuminemia due to protein loss from the gastric mucosa.

Prognosis

Most patients survive up to 5 to 10 years after diagnosis of carcinoid tumor.

Treatment

Octreotide, a somatostatin analog, is the standard treatment for carcinoid tumor. It inhibits gut hormone release and consequently stops the flushing and diarrhea. Inhibition of tumor growth can occur in some patients. Some tumors secrete other hormones, producing different clinical syndromes (e.g., adrenocorticotropic hormone excess resulting in Cushing's syndrome). Consequently, treatment should be tailored to the manifestations.

Peutz-Jeghers syndrome

Clinical features

Mucocutaneous pigmentation of the face, hands, and feet with multiple polyps along the intestine. The polyps can manifest with bleeding and occasionally intussusception.

Diagnosis and evaluation

Barium enema or barium follow-through is carried out to demonstrate the extent of polyposis with confirmation by biopsy taken at colonoscopy or enteroscopy.

Etiology and pathogenesis

Peutz-Jeghers syndrome is inherited as an autosomal dominant trait. The polyps are hamartomas and can occur anywhere along the GI tract, but they occur particularly in the small bowel.

Complications

There is a small but definite risk of malignant change of hamartomas involved in Peutz-Jeghers syndrome.

Treatment

Polypectomies should be carried out along the bowel to look for dysplastic features, but bowel resection should be avoided if possible. Regular endoscopic and histologic surveillance is necessary, the frequency of which can be guided by the grade of dysplasia.

Bacterial overgrowth

Clinical features

Malabsorption (i.e., diarrhea, steatorrhea, and vitamin deficiency, especially B_{12}) tends to be the predominant feature of bacterial overgrowth.

Diagnosis and evaluation

Investigations of value include:

- Hydrogen breath test. Oral lactulose or glucose is ingested and metabolized by the bacteria to hydrogen, which can be detected in expiration (see Fig. 24.8). However, interpretation can be difficult because there are bacteria present in the oral cavity, and rapid transit time will allow bacteria in the large intestine to break down lactulose.
- ^{14}C-glycocholic acid breath test. ^{14}C-labeled bile salt is ingested, and bacteria deconjugate the bile salts and release $^{14}CO_2$, which can be detected in exhaled breath. Rapid transit time will also cause a rise in radioactivity due to substrate reaching bacteria in the large intestines.
- Small intestinal aspiration. Direct aspiration followed by aerobic and anaerobic cultures can be an alternative method for diagnosing bacterial overgrowth.

Etiology and pathogenesis

Gastric acid normally kills most bacteria, and intestinal motility keeps the jejunum free of bacteria. The terminal ileum usually contains fecal type of bacteria (e.g., *Escherichia coli*, *Enterococcus* species, and anaerobes such as *Bacteroides* species).

Bacterial overgrowth occurs as a result of structural abnormality (i.e., Polya gastrectomy, small intestinal diverticulosis, strictures, or where stasis exists), allowing bacteria to grow. The condition can also be seen in elderly persons and in scleroderma (due to hypomotility).

Deconjugation of bile salts by the bacteria can result in fat malabsorption (i.e., steatorrhea) and deficiency of the fat-soluble vitamins A, D, E, and K. The bacteria can also metabolize vitamin B_{12} and interfere with its binding to intrinsic factor, causing vitamin B_{12} deficiency. Folate levels tend to be elevated consequent on bacterial metabolism.

 Patients with vitamin B_{12} deficiency due to bacterial overgrowth often have a high serum folate level due to its absorption after production by the bacteria.

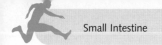

Complications

Complications result from malabsorption of vitamin B_{12} and fat-soluble vitamins, causing macrocytic anemia, peripheral neuropathy (rarely), osteomalacia, coagulopathy, etc.

Treatment

Treatment of the underlying cause (e.g., strictures, blind loop in Polya gastrectomy) should be addressed and may require surgical resection. Multiple diverticula and other conditions may not be amenable to surgery. Prolonged or cyclical courses of antibiotics are usually required in an attempt to reestablish normal intestinal flora. Antibacterial agents such as metronidazole and tetracycline or ciprofloxacin are found to be effective. Vitamin deficiency should be corrected.

Tropical sprue
Clinical features

The clinical features of tropical sprue include:
- Diarrhea, with malabsorption and nutritional deficiency.
- Weight loss.
- Anorexia.

Diagnosis is reserved for persons resident in epidemic areas such as Asia, South America, and parts of the Caribbean. Often there is a preceding enteric infection.

Diagnosis and evaluation

Investigations to aid in the diagnosis of tropical sprue include the following:
- Stool culture is necessary to exclude other causes of infective diarrhea (e.g., giardiasis).
- Jejunal biopsy shows partial villous atrophy, but it is usually less severe than that of celiac disease.

Etiology and pathogenesis

There is likely to be an infective cause present in tropical sprue, but the exact etiology is unknown. A number of pathogens have been implicated, but conclusive evidence is unavailable. There could be geographic variation with differing precipitants from country to country.

Complications

Folate deficiency is common. Complications are a result of vitamin deficiency seen in any malabsorptive state.

Treatment

An improvement of symptoms is frequently seen corresponding with departure from the endemic area.

Most patients will require antibiotics (e.g., tetracycline) for up to 6 months. Folic acid and other vitamin supplements are also required.

Whipple's disease
Incidence

Whipple's disease occurs rarely and particularly affects middle-aged men.

Clinical features

The clinical features of Whipple's disease include:
- Steatorrhea.
- Abdominal pain.
- Fever.
- Weight loss.

Peripheral lymphadenopathy, migratory arthritis, and pigmentation may also be seen.

Involvement of the brain causes chronic encephalitis and may be the dominant feature.

Diagnosis and evaluation

Jejunal biopsy typically demonstrates the cells of the lamina propria replaced with periodic acid–Schiff–positive macrophages, which represent the remains of dead bacteria. There is usually only minimal villous atrophy.

Etiology and pathogenesis

The bacteria responsible have been identified as *Tropheryma whippelii* and are thought to be of low infectivity. The exact mechanism of the disease is uncertain but may involve a type of immunodeficiency.

Treatment

Prolonged antibiotic therapy with agents such as penicillin, tetracycline, or chloramphenicol, is effective and improvement can be dramatic. Supplements of relevant vitamins and minerals may be required for patients with severe malabsorption.

Tuberculosis
Incidence

TB is rare in the United States but should be suspected in areas where it is more common (e.g., Asia) and in the context of known HIV infection.

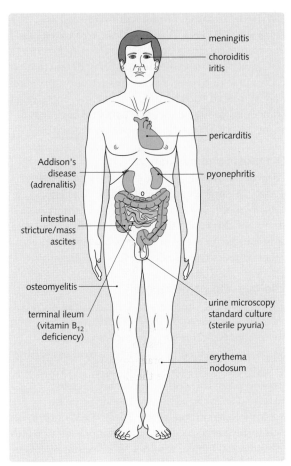

Fig. 16.6 Body map of features seen in extrapulmonary TB.

Clinical features

The clinical features of TB are similar to those of Crohn's disease (e.g., weight loss, abdominal pain, anorexia, anemia) (Fig. 16.6). Intestinal obstruction may occur. A right iliac fossa mass may be palpable. It can also manifest as tuberculous (exudative) ascites, which may mimic malignant disease. Vitamin B_{12} deficiency may exist as a result of terminal ileal involvement.

Diagnosis and evaluation

Consider the following methods to diagnose:

- Abdominal ultrasound may show mesenteric thickening and lymph node involvement.
- Laparotomy for histologic confirmation followed by bacteriologic confirmation is the gold standard, but TB cultures can take up to 6 weeks.
- Chest radiograph may demonstrate evidence of coexistent pulmonary TB and thus aid in the diagnosis of small intestine TB.

Etiology and pathogenesis

TB usually occurs as a consequence of reactivation of the primary disease caused by *Mycobacterium tuberculosis*. Bovine TB is very rare and is due to ingestion of unpasteurized milk. The ileocecal area is most commonly affected. Typical caseating granulomas are seen histologically.

Treatment

Similar antibacterial agents are used as they are for pulmonary TB (e.g., triple therapy of isoniazid, rifampin, and pyrazinamide). Treatment is often extended for at least 9 months.

Yersinia infection
Clinical features

In adults, *Yersinia* infection causes an enterocolitis characterized by fever, diarrhea, and abdominal pain. It can also give rise to terminal ileitis, which often clinically is mistaken for appendicitis.

Reiter's syndrome (conjunctivitis, arthritis, and nonspecific urethritis) can sometimes occur after infection with *Yersinia* organisms. Manifestations such as erythema nodosum and seronegative arthritis are not uncommon and are probably related to circulating immune complexes.

In children, the infection is more likely to cause mesenteric adenitis, giving rise to abdominal pain.

Diagnosis

Diagnosis is not routinely confirmed but is occasionally made on tissue diagnosis or lymph node biopsy (e.g., after appendectomy).

Etiology and pathogenesis

The offending organisms are *Y. enterocolitica* (enterocolitis) and *Y. pseudotuberculosis* (terminal ileitis).

Treatment

Yersinia infection is usually a self-limiting disease, and no specific treatment may be necessary. In severe cases, tetracycline may be given.

Giardiasis
Incidence

Giardiasis is common in the tropics and is an important cause of traveler's diarrhea.

Clinical features

Typical symptoms include:

99

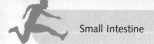

- Watery (nonbloody) diarrhea.
- Nausea.
- Anorexia.
- Abdominal pain.
- Malabsorption and disaccharide intolerance may occur.

Asymptomatic carriage is also observed.

Diagnosis and evaluation
Stool examination is important, but cysts can be seen only in fresh stool samples because they often die when stored.

Negative stool examination results do not exclude the diagnosis because excretion of the parasite can be intermittent.

Duodenal aspirate or biopsy allows direct visualization of the parasite. Serology-specific IgG and IgM antibodies can be measured.

Etiology and pathogenesis
Giardia lamblia is a flagellate protozoan that is found worldwide, and epidemics have been reported in parts of Europe and North America.

Transmission is by the fecal-oral route and mainly via contaminated water supplies.

The organism colonizes within the small intestinal wall and can produce an asymptomatic infection. However, in most cases villous atrophy ensues, causing diarrhea and malabsorption.

The exact mechanism by which *Giardia* organisms cause villous atrophy is unknown, but an immune-mediated response may be responsible. Bacterial overgrowth may account for some of the malabsorption seen.

Complications
Complications are mainly due to malabsorption of vitamins and malnutrition seen in small bowel disease. If diarrhea persists, consider lactose intolerance and recommend a trial of abstinence from milk.

Treatment
Metronidazole is the drug of choice given for 7 to 10 days with or without vitamin supplements.

Cholera
Clinical features
The incubation period of cholera can range from a few hours to 6 days.

Diarrhea is often profuse and watery (also painless). It is classically likened to "rice water" stool due to presence of mucus.

Circulatory collapse due to profound dehydration occurs in severe cases. As much as 1 L of watery stool may be passed each hour. Consequently, acute renal failure and profound electrolyte disturbance may ensue.

Diagnosis and evaluation
Diagnosis is mainly made on clinical grounds.

Stool examination is helpful. The flagellate, actively motile organism can be seen in freshly passed stool, but this is not specific for cholera, as a similar appearance can occur in *Campylobacter* infections. Stool cultures will usually confirm the diagnosis.

Etiology and pathogenesis
Transmission of the gram-negative bacillus *Vibrio cholerae* is achieved by the fecal-oral route via contaminated water supplies and food sources. Exotoxins produced by the bacteria bind irreversibly to epithelial receptors along the small intestine that activate adenylate cyclase and hence increase intracellular cyclic adenosine monophosphate (cAMP) concentrations (Fig. 16.7). This, in turn, causes the stimulation of salt and water secretion into the intestinal lumen, resulting in a devastating loss of fluid and electrolytes. Reabsorption of fluid in the small intestine is also inhibited, contributing to the fluid loss.

Treatment
Fluid and electrolyte replacement, either intravenously or orally, is the mainstay of treatment.

Antibiotics such as tetracycline will shorten the duration of the illness, but drug resistance is an increasing problem. Oral vaccines (live and killed) are emerging as effective preventive measures.

Strongyloidiasis
Clinical features
Typical symptoms include:
- Local skin erythema and itching where the larvae have gained entry.
- Respiratory symptoms, such as cough and (rarely) pneumonitis, approximately 7 to 10 days after initial penetration.
- Abdominal discomfort, intermittent diarrhea, and constipation seen approximately 3 weeks later, when intestinal colonization occurs. Heavy

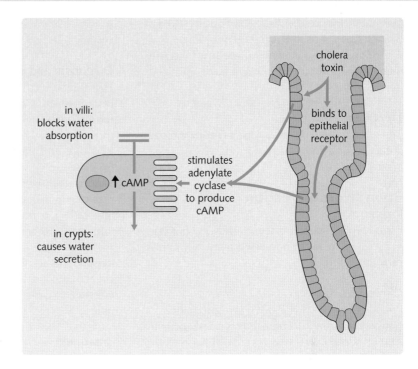

Fig. 16.7 Mechanisms of diarrhea in cholera infection.

infestation may result in more marked manifestations, including steatorrhea and intestinal malabsorption.

Diagnosis and evaluation
An eosinophilia is commonly revealed by a complete blood count.

Larvae can be detected in fresh stool sample or duodenal aspirate.

Etiology and pathogenesis
Strongyloidiasis is caused by infection with *Strongyloides stercoralis*, found especially in South America and Asia. Infection can persist for decades, and new cases are still diagnosed in war veterans who were infected while abroad.

Adult worms reside in the crypts of the small intestine, provoking an inflammatory response with consequent mucosal damage. The worms are excreted in the stool, and autoinfection is common.

Complications
Disseminated strongyloidiasis is a rare but often fatal condition seen in persons who are immunocompromised.

Treatment
Thiabendazole or albendazole (fewer side effects) provides effective treatment.

Hookworm infection
Incidence
Hookworm infection is seen worldwide and is said to affect one quarter of the world's population.

Clinical features
Clinical features include:
- Local skin irritation where the worm gains entry.
- Mild respiratory symptoms seen approximately 2 weeks later.
- Iron-deficiency anemia.

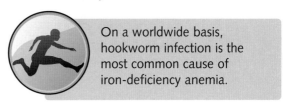

On a worldwide basis, hookworm infection is the most common cause of iron-deficiency anemia.

Diagnosis and evaluation
Complete blood count shows a microcytic hypochromic anemia. Eosinophilia may be seen early in the course of the infection. Microscopy can demonstrate ova in a fresh stool sample.

Etiology and pathogenesis
Ancylostoma duodenale is responsible for the cases found in Europe and Middle East, whereas *Necator*

101

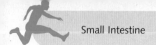

americanus causes the disease in Southeast Asia, the Far East, and sub-Saharan Africa.

The adult worm attaches to the small intestinal mucosa by its buccal capsule and feeds off blood from the mucosa.

Treatment
The treatment of choice is mebendazole, a broad-spectrum anthelminthic that is effective against hookworms.

Roundworm infection
Incidence
Roundworm infection is seen worldwide but is particularly prevalent in socioeconomically deprived, rural areas.

Clinical features
Roundworm infection is often asymptomatic. Nausea, vomiting, abdominal discomfort, diarrhea, and intestinal obstruction occur with heavy infections.

Invasion of the appendix or biliary tree will cause appendicitis and biliary obstruction, respectively.

Larvae in the lung will cause pulmonary eosinophilia.

Diagnosis and evaluation
Eggs can be seen on microscopic preparations taken from fresh stool samples. Adult worms may appear from the mouth or anus.

Etiology and pathogenesis
Roundworm infection is caused by *Ascaris lumbricoides*, which can grow to a considerable size, resulting in malnutrition in some cases. Eggs are ingested via a fecally contaminated source and hatch into larvae in the small intestine. They can travel via the portal system to the liver and lungs, where they develop further. Pulmonary larvae may be expectorated and then swallowed back into the intestine to grow into mature worms up to 20 inches in length.

Treatment
Mebendazole is effective against the parasite. Surgical intervention may be needed for acute appendicitis and intestinal obstruction.

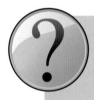

- What are the mechanisms that facilitate absorption of nutrients through the intestinal mucosa?
- What are the systemic manifestations of Crohn's disease?
- What investigations should be performed for a patient with an acute exacerbation of Crohn's disease?
- What maintenance pharmacologic therapies should be considered in the treatment of patients with frequently relapsing Crohn's disease?
- What are the clinical features of celiac disease?
- What are the potential complications of bacterial overgrowth?
- Describe the mechanism of diarrhea in cholera infection.

Ulcerative colitis vs. Crohn's disease		
	Ulcerative colitis	Crohn's disease
Clinical features	Bloody diarrhea	Abdominal pain and weight loss
Macroscopic appearance	Usually confined to colon Rectum always involved Ulceration superficial and continuous	Most often terminal ileum but can affect anywhere in GI tract Patchy transmural ulceration and skip lesions are common
Microscopic appearance	Crypt abscesses	Granulomas are common

Fig. 17.5 Contrasting features between ulcerative colitis and Crohn's disease.

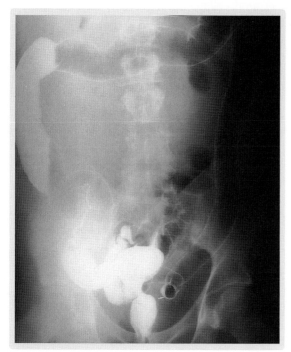

Fig. 17.6 Barium enema showing "lead-pipe" appearance in chronic ulcerative colitis.

Complications

Toxic megacolon is seen on plain abdominal radiograph. Dilatation of 5 cm or greater is associated with a risk of perforation and peritonitis. The patient is usually unwell with fever, tachycardia, and abdominal distention with tenderness (Figs. 17.2 and 17.7). Shock with oliguric renal failure can occur as a consequence of sepsis and hypovolemia.

The risk of developing adenocarcinoma after 10 years of colitis is approximately 5% higher than in the general population. The risk is related to the extent of colon involved and the duration of the disease process. The current recommendations for screening in this regard are as follows:

Features of severe ulcerative colitis
Stool frequency >8 times/day with blood
Abdominal pain and tenderness
Fever >37.5°C
Tachycardia >100 bpm
C-reactive protein >20 mg/L ESR >35 mm/h
Hemoglobin <10 g/L
Albumin <30 g/L

Fig. 17.7 Features indicating severity in ulcerative colitis (ESR, erthrocyte sedimentation rate).

- The initial screen should occur at 8 years for those with pancolitis and for left-sided colitis, 15 years from onset of symptoms.
- Colonoscopy (with biopsy specimens taken every 10 cm) should be performed every 3 years in the second decade, every 2 years in the third decade, and annually thereafter.
- Hemorrhage is a potential complication, although blood transfusion is usually required only in severe attacks.
- Cholangiocarcinoma arises with increasing frequency in patients with ulcerative colitis when primary sclerosing cholangitis coexists.
- Secondary amyloidosis is probably related to high levels of circulating acute-phase protein during exacerbations.

 Abdominal pain in ulcerative colitis is an ominous feature and may indicate development of toxic megacolon or perforation.

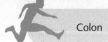

Prognosis

The course of ulcerative colitis is variable, but characteristically it is a chronic relapsing disease. Patients with proctitis alone have a good overall prognosis, with only 10% progressing to more extensive disease. By contrast, severe fulminant disease is associated with a mortality rate of up to 25%.

Treatment

Treatment options include:

- Corticosteroids given during an acute attack to gain remission. Topical treatment can be given for localized disease (e.g., proctitis) in the form of an enema. Long-term use of oral steroids should be avoided.
- The management of an acute, severe attack may necessitate intravenous steroids (e.g., hydrocortisone), intravenous fluid and electrolyte replacement, and appropriate antibiotics for proven or suspected coexistent infection. Intravenous nutrition (i.e., total parenteral nutrition) may be required for protracted exacerbations, and intramuscular vitamins are sometimes given.
- 5-Aminosalicylic acid (5-ASA) compounds are effective in reducing acute inflammation and maintaining remission in ulcerative colitis. Sulfasalazine is attached to sulfapyridine, which is broken down by bacteria to active 5-ASA. Mesalazine (5-ASA alone) or olsalazine (two 5-ASA moieties) may be less toxic because they do not have a sulfur compound conjugated. These can also be given in enema form for localized proctitis.
- Immunosuppression with azathioprine can be used for patients who are not responding to steroids or in frequently relapsing cases where long-term steroid use is undesirable. Azathioprine is an antiproliferative immunosuppressant with the rare but serious adverse effect of myelosuppression. Blood counts should be monitored closely for the first few weeks, and the patient should be warned to report immediately any signs or symptoms of bone marrow suppression (e.g., infections, bleeding, or spontaneous bruising). Hepatic toxicity is also well recognized.
- Surgical resection, usually in form of colectomy, is imperative for patients with complications such as toxic megacolon or perforation and may be required in patients not responding to medical treatment. Total surgical mortality rates are approximately 5%, and in the acute situation with perforation, they can be as high as 50%.

Crohn's colitis

Clinical features

Crohn's disease can affect any part of the intestine, including the colon, and is occasionally confined to the colon alone (i.e., Crohn's colitis).

It can be difficult to differentiate Crohn's colitis from ulcerative colitis, and the two conditions can overlap (a condition referred to as "indeterminate colitis").

The clinical picture is of abdominal pain and diarrhea. Pain is more common in Crohn's colitis than in ulcerative colitis, and bleeding is far less common.

Evaluation and diagnosis

Evaluation and diagnosis for Crohn's colitis are basically the same as for ulcerative colitis. Differentiation from ulcerative colitis can be difficult.

The presence of granulomas and deep inflammation is suggestive of Crohn's colitis, whereas paucity of mucin and crypt abscesses are more in favor of ulcerative colitis.

Etiology and pathogenesis

Up to 15% of patients with Crohn's colitis will have clinical features of ulcerative colitis, but the biopsy will reveal the presence of granulomas, which are pathognomonic of Crohn's disease, therefore making the diagnosis difficult.

Recent genetic studies have shown that a presence of certain genes occurring simultaneously predisposes a person to developing inflammatory bowel disease. It is now thought that ulcerative colitis and Crohn's disease may represent opposite ends of a spectrum.

Treatment

Standard treatment remains the same. However, it is important to distinguish between Crohn's and ulcerative colitis because there are important implications in their treatment. For example, surgery is generally considered to be curative in ulcerative colitis, whereas this is clearly not the case for Crohn's disease.

See Chapter 16 for further details on Crohn's disease.

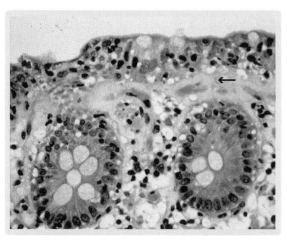

Fig. 17.8 Photomicrograph of collagenous colitis. Note the thickened amorphous layer just below the surface epithelial cells (arrow).

Collagenous colitis
Clinical features
Collagenous colitis occurs more commonly in women and presents as intermittent chronic watery diarrhea. Abdominal pain may also be present. Patients are asymptomatic during remission.

Diagnosis and evaluation
Stool culture, inflammatory markers, and colonoscopy usually compose the normal testing process.

Diagnosis is based on histology, which demonstrates the presence of a thickened subepithelial collagen layer (Fig. 17.8). There may also be intraepithelial lymphocytic infiltration, but this is more commonly seen in microscopic colitis (see below).

Etiology and pathogenesis
There is an association with long-term use of nonsteroidal anti-inflammatory drugs (NSAIDs), but an underlying immunologic cause has been postulated because this condition is more commonly seen in persons with seronegative arthritis, Raynaud's phenomenon, and celiac disease.

Treatment
The use of NSAIDs should be stopped. Antidiarrheal drugs are ineffective. Sulfasalazine and cholestyramine have been tried with variable success rates. In persistent cases, short-term oral corticosteroids can be employed.

Microscopic colitis
Clinical features
The typical symptoms of microscopic colitis are similar to those of collagenous colitis (e.g., intermittent diarrhea, abdominal pain). Again, the condition is more commonly found in women.

Diagnosis and evaluation
The diagnosis and evaluation for microscopic colitis are the same as for collagenous colitis, except the biopsy shows intraepithelial lymphocytic infiltration without thickening of the collagen layer.

Etiology and pathogenesis
An immune etiology has also been suggested because there is an association with:
• Increased frequency of patients who have HLA-A1 haplotype.
• Decreased frequency of HLA-A3.

In addition, a minority of patients with microscopic colitis have subsequently been found to have celiac disease.

Treatment
Recommended treatment for microscopic colitis is the same as for collagenous colitis. Cholestyramine may also be helpful.

Neoplastic disorders

Colonic polyps
Clinical features
Usually, colonic polyps are an incidental finding as part of an investigation for abdominal pain, rectal bleeding, altered bowel habit, etc. In addition:
• Obstruction and intussusception can occur, especially in infants.
• Iron-deficiency anemia may be present if the polyp ulcerates or bleeds.
• Diarrhea is seen with the villous type and can be severe enough to cause hypokalemia.

Diagnosis and evaluation
Appropriate tests include:
• Barium enema, which may demonstrate either solitary or multiple polyps.
• Endoscopy, which is used to confirm and remove polyps for histologic examination (see Fig. 24.21).

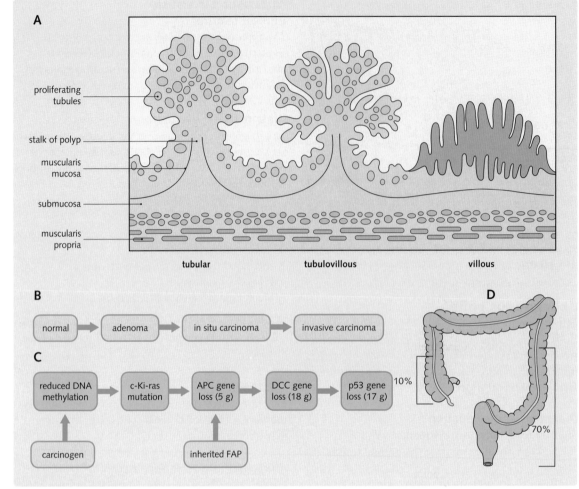

Fig. 17.9 A. Types of colonic polyps. B. A summary of the polyp cancer sequence in the colon. C. Molecular changes involved. D. Two thirds of colon cancers occur within 60 cm of the anal verge and within reach of a flexible sigmoidoscope (FAP, familial adenomatous polyposis).

Etiology and pathogenesis

The majority of polyps are adenomas (tubular, tubulovillous, or villous).

The malignant potential of any polyp is related to:
- Increasing polyp size.
- Polyp type (i.e., tubulovillous rather than metaplastic) (Fig. 17.9).

Polyps can be solitary or multiple. Genetic and environmental factors have been implicated because they are more commonly seen in the Western world (10% of the population), but no definite cause has been found. Almost all colonic carcinomas originate from a polyp, and 90% of patients with colonic carcinoma will have polyps elsewhere in the colon. Five percent of polyps removed at sigmoidoscopies are found to have invasive carcinoma.

Familial polyposis coli is an inherited autosomal dominant condition involving a gene located on the long arm of chromosome 5. There are polyps throughout the gastrointestinal (GI) tract, especially in the colon, and patients commonly present with this condition while in their teens. Hypertrophy and osteomas of the mandibles and long bones are commonly associated with this syndrome.

The other main type of polyps is the hamartoma, such as in Peutz-Jeghers syndrome (see Chapter 16). More common in children are juvenile polyps, which histologically are shown to be mucus-retention cysts and are mainly confined to the colon.

Persons who have Cronkhite-Canada syndrome have polyps similar to those of Peutz-Jeghers syndrome, but in addition they have ectodermal abnormalities such as nail dystrophy and skin pigmentation.

Complications
Complication of colonic polyps include:
- Malignant change with increasing size.
- Bleeding, obstruction, and intussusception.

Prognosis
There is a 50% chance of recurrence after the removal of an adenomatous polyp.

Treatment
Treatment involves:
- Endoscopic removal of polyps. Any lesions found on endoscopy or barium studies should ideally be removed to prevent malignant transformation (see Fig. 24.18).
- Surgical resection for patients with familial polyposis coli, for whom individual polyps cannot be removed.
- Surveillance of patients who are at risk (e.g., those with polyposis coli and their first-degree relatives).
- Colonoscopic screening for those who have had a colonic adenoma, undertaken according to the size and number of polyps (assigned low, intermediate, or high risk). For example, one or two adenomas measuring less than 1 cm in diameter may only need one screen after 5 years, whereas multiple large polyps require annual colonoscopy.

Always be alerted by a history of sustained change in bowel habit, particularly in persons older than 45 years of age. Colonic carcinoma should be excluded in this setting.

Colorectal carcinoma
Incidence
The second most common carcinoma in the United States, colorectal carcinoma affects approximately 20 of every 100,000 persons. The mean age at diagnosis is between 60 and 65 years. The disease is rare in Africa and Asia and this is thought to be linked to environmental rather than genetic factors.

Etiology and pathogenesis
Western diets of high animal fat and low fiber have been linked to colorectal carcinoma, possibly due to slow transit of intestinal content, which increases contact time between potential carcinogens and the bowel wall.

Familial polyposis coli and inflammatory bowel disease are risk factors for the development of colonic tumors. The relationship between inflammatory bowel disease and carcinomas is not clearly defined, but it does not appear to be directly associated with chronicity of inflammation. It is possible that the risk for development of colonic carcinoma is an inherited one because the age of onset is more important than the severity of the disease and seems to be an independent risk factor.

Colonic carcinoma is now thought to be a result of multiple genetic alterations that occur in a progressive, stepwise manner. Oncogenes that normally regulate cell division and differentiation may undergo mutation as a result of external stimuli. This produces hyperplasia, followed by metaplasia, and eventually dysplastic change and tumor. Most commonly associated with colonic carcinoma are the c-KRAS and c-MYC oncogenes. The APC gene on the long arm of chromosome 5 is responsible for familial polyposis coli, which may have a role in development of colonic carcinoma (see Fig. 17.9).

Dukes' classification of colonic cancer is shown in Fig. 17.10.

Hereditary colonic carcinomas have been described, and the gene responsible is located on chromosome 2. These patients have tumors at an early age (i.e., peak incidence at 40 years) and typically have a right-sided lesion (i.e., Lynch syndrome type I). Some of these patients also have an increased incidence of other carcinomas, such as endometrial, brain, and lung, as well as other GI tract carcinomas (i.e., Lynch syndrome type II).

Approximately two thirds of tumors arise from the rectosigmoid colon, and these tumors typically start off as a flat lesion and later become bulky, polypoid, and ulcerate. Similar types of lesions are found in the cecum and ascending colon. Lesions in the descending colon tend to be annular and produce the typical "apple core" lesion on barium enema (see Fig. 24.25).

The tumors produce a variable amount of mucin, and histologically signet ring cells can be seen where the nucleus is pushed to one side due to cytoplasmic mucus.

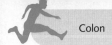

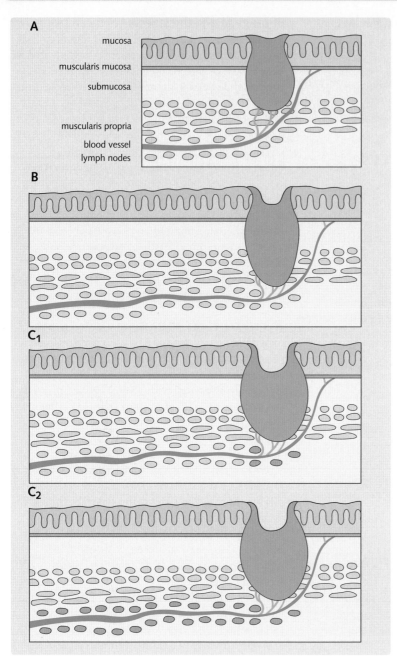

Fig. 17.10 Dukes' classification of colonic cancer. A. The tumor invades muscularis propria but not serosa. B. The tumor extends through the muscle coat into serosa nodes but not lymph nodes. C. All layers are affected (transmural invasion and lymph nodes), with the proximal lymph node affected in C_1 and both the proximal and the highest resected nodes positive in C_2.

Clinical features

The main features of colorectal carcinoma are as follows:

- Anemia, weight loss, abdominal pain, or loose bowel motions are the most common features. A mass may be palpable in the right iliac fossa, especially with cecal lesions. Rectal bleeding or obstruction is more common with left-sided lesions (e.g., rectosigmoid).
- Altered bowel habits are seen in more than 50% of all patients.
- Perforation and abscess formation are not uncommon, and jaundice due to liver metastases can occur in advanced cases.

Rectal examination is a mandatory part of the examination because a tumor can often be palpated.

Diagnosis and evaluation

Tests of use include:

- Complete blood count. This may detect iron-deficiency anemia, which is common.
- Fecal occult blood, which often has positive results but can be seen in any cause of underlying GI tract bleed (e.g., duodenal ulceration).
- Barium enema, which is still the investigation of choice in most centers. Poor bowel preparation can make interpretation difficult.
- Flexible sigmoidoscopy. This test can detect up to 70% of tumors and is better in combination with barium enema to examine the remainder of the colon. Colonoscopy is reserved for patients unsuitable for barium enema or in doubtful cases. Adequate bowel preparation is essential.
- Abdominal ultrasound, which is sensitive for detecting metastases in the liver before surgical resection.

Treatment

The mainstays of management are:

- Surgical resection with end-to-end anastomosis or end colostomy, depending on the site of the tumor.
- Chemotherapy with or without radiotherapy, given to patients with Dukes' B and C disease (see Fig. 17.10) and can improve survival. Chemotherapy is administered to patients with liver metastases.

Prognosis

The overall survival rate of colorectal carcinoma is 30% at 5 years (Fig. 17.11).

Angiodysplasia

Incidence

Angiodysplasia is a relatively rare condition affecting the elderly population.

Clinical features

Features of angiodysplasia to note are as follows:

- Chronic iron-deficiency anemia is due to chronic blood loss from the GI tract.

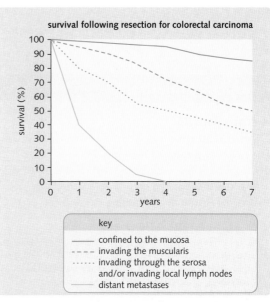

Fig. 17.11 Survival after resection for colorectal carcinoma, according to Dukes' staging. Note that survival is commensurate with that of the normal population if the tumor is confined to the mucosa.

- Acute GI tract bleeding can occur, causing hypotension and shock in some patients.

Diagnosis and evaluation

Diagnosis of angiodysplasia can be difficult and often involves repeated gastroscopy and colonoscopy to detect the lesion:

- Red-cell radioisotope-labeled scanning can be helpful to identify the site of blood loss.
- Selective angiography may demonstrate abnormal blood vessels or the site of active bleeding.

Etiology and pathogenesis

The underlying etiology of angiodysplasia is unknown, but the condition is most likely to be acquired because it mainly affects the elderly population. There is an association with aortic stenosis, and approximately half of the patients will have some form of cardiac disease. It can exist anywhere along the GI tract but is more commonly found in the proximal colon, cecum, and terminal ileum.

Treatment

Diathermy during colonoscopy can be successful for small lesions. Larger proximal lesions will need

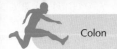
surgical resection. Hormonal treatment with progesterone derivatives can result in the regression of the lesions.

Anorectal conditions

Hemorrhoids
Clinical features
The main symptoms of hemorrhoids are:
- Rectal bleeding, which may coat the stools or drip into the toilet at the end of defecation.
- Perianal irritation and itching.

 Bleeding from hemorrhoids is bright red. This is because it is capillary blood from the spongy vascular anal cushions. Hemorrhoids are not "varicose veins."

Diagnosis and evaluation
Proctoscopy reveals blood vessels classically seen at the 3-, 7-, and 11-o'clock positions.

Etiology and pathogenesis
Hemorrhoids result from enlargement of the venous plexuses at the lower end of anal mucosa.

Raised intra-abdominal pressure inhibits venous return to the vena cava and hence causes venous engorgement. Common contributing factors are constipation, pregnancy, and excessive straining to pass urine or stool.

A minor degree of rectal prolapse is common. Estrogen-related venous dilatation may also contribute to the development of hemorrhoids in pregnancy.

Rectal bleeding occurs as a result of trauma by passage of hard stools. Symptoms are usually intermittent and exacerbated by constipation.

Mucus secreted by glandular epithelium can block skin pores, which causes secondary infection by bacteria and *Candida* organisms, followed by local skin irritation. Hemorrhoids are classified as first, second, and third degree, as shown in Fig. 17.12. They may be painful if they thrombose.

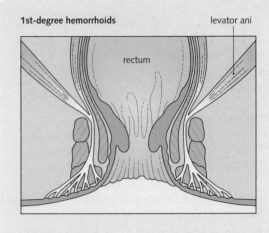

1st-degree hemorrhoids   levator ani

rectum

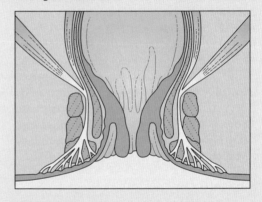

2nd-degree hemorrhoids

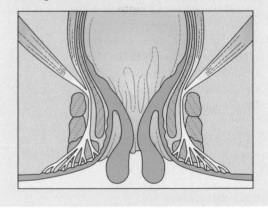

3rd-degree hemorrhoids

Fig. 17.12 Anatomic representation of hemorrhoid classification. In first-degree hemorrhoids, the spongy vascular cushions remain within the rectum. Second-degree hemorrhoids prolapse through the anus on defecation but spontaneously reduce, whereas third-degree hemorrhoids require digital reduction or may remain persistently prolapsed.

Complications

Thrombosis of the hemorrhoids is painful and irreducible. However, it is a self-limiting condition that eventually results in atrophy and fibrosis of the thrombosed hemorrhoids, leaving visible anal tags.

Treatment

Mild cases of hemorrhoids can be improved simply by addressing the underlying constipation; a high-fiber diet may be all that is necessary.

- Injection of a sclerosant or elastic band ligation may be needed in more troublesome cases.
- Surgical resection is reserved for irreducible, prolapsed, and problematic cases.

Anal fissures
Clinical features

Rectal pain during defecation associated with rectal bleeding is the classic presentation of anal fissures. Pain, in turn, will cause anal spasm and aggravate the constipation that caused the condition originally.

Diagnosis

A diagnosis of anal fissures is often made on clinical grounds. Rectal examination is extremely painful and rarely possible. If rectal examination is required, local or general anesthesia may be used.

A small skin tag or sentinel pile may be seen at the anus, and parting of the buttocks may reveal the fissure itself.

Etiology and pathogenesis

Anal fissures are usually the result of the passage of a large constipated stool causing a tear in the anal mucosa. Over 90% of cases are in the midline of the posterior margin and are perpetuated by internal sphincter spasm.

Treatment

Treatment depends on the type of fissure:

- Acute fissures can be treated with local anesthesia and prevention of further constipation with either a bulking agent or osmotic laxative.
- Chronic fissuring may require surgical intervention in the form of anal stretch or, more recently introduced, lateral internal sphincterotomy, which has a better result with regard to incontinence in later age. Glyceryl trinitrate ointment can improve pain and ischemia caused by chronic fissuring and spasm and may negate the need for surgery.

Pruritus ani

Pruritus ani is a common complaint. The majority of cases result from poor hygiene and some degree of fecal incontinence, especially in elderly persons. Associated conditions such as hemorrhoids, threadworm infestation, or fungal infection should be excluded.

In the absence of any underlying cause, treatment should include good personal hygiene and keeping the area dry. Use of topical steroids or antimicrobial creams should be avoided.

Rectal prolapse
Incidence

Rectal prolapse is common among elderly persons and young children.

Clinical features

Tenesmus is a feeling of incomplete defecation, which can be due to prolapse. Rectal bleeding can occur due to mucosal ulceration resulting from stool trauma. Incontinence of feces may be seen.

Complete prolapse of the rectal wall can sometimes be seen through the anus (Fig. 17.13).

Diagnosis and evaluation

Diagnosis of rectal prolapse is usually made based on history and examination. However:

- Sigmoidoscopy may reveal a "solitary" rectal ulcer approximately 8 to 10 cm above the anal verge, usually on the anterior rectal wall. These solitary ulcers can also be multiple.
- Prolapse can often be seen when the patient is asked to voluntarily strain as if to pass a stool.
- A defecating proctogram is a very useful, albeit undignified, examination if the prolapse is internal but producing significant symptoms.
- Endoscopic ultrasound can be useful to determine whether muscle damage has occurred (possibly due to obstetric trauma) because this condition can be repaired surgically.

Etiology and pathogenesis

Rectal prolapse results from excessive straining when opening bowels. In the initial stages, the

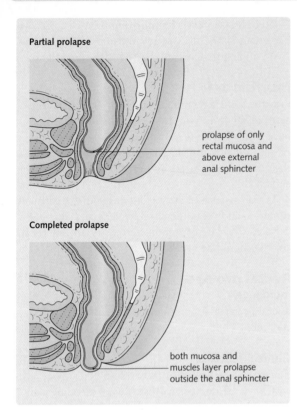

Fig. 17.13 Classification of rectal prolapse.

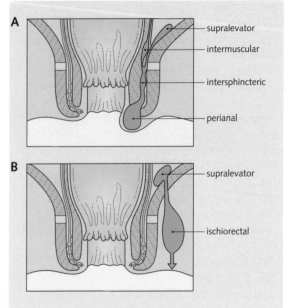

Fig. 17.14 The process by which perianal infection can develop into abscess (A) or fistula (B).

prolapse occurs only after defecation and returns spontaneously, but later the condition worsens and prolapse may appear on standing.

In early stages, prolapse of the mucosa or rectal wall may remain internal to the anal sphincter; hence, the patient may experience discomfort but no obvious abnormality can be seen.

Treatment

Rectal prolapse in childhood rarely requires surgical treatment. Parents should be reassured because the prolapse will almost always be reduced either spontaneously or with gentle manipulation. A high-fiber diet should be given, and the child should be taught not to strain at defecation.

Minor prolapses often do not require treatment because they reduce themselves and appear only after straining. General advice such as adopting a high-fiber diet and avoidance of straining should be given. Patients with severe prolapse should be treated surgically by posterior fixation of the rectum to the sacral wall. Sphincter repair may also be necessary if problematic incontinence occurs as a result of a weakened sphincter.

Anorectal abscesses
Clinical features

Pain depends upon the site of an anorectal abscess:
- A fluctuant mass sitting just beneath the inflamed skin is typical of perianal and ischiorectal abscesses.
- A tender mass on rectal examination may be due to intersphincteric or pararectal abscesses.

Systemic features of infection such as fever and neutrophilia may occur.

Etiology and pathogenesis

Anorectal abscesses are more often seen in patients with diabetes, Crohn's disease, and conditions or therapies leading to immunosuppression, but they do occur in otherwise healthy persons. The condition is due to infection of the anal glands, which tends to spread along the anal duct through the external sphincter and its surrounding tissues (Fig. 17.14).

Treatment

Surgical drainage is required in all cases, except for those that are very minor—for these, antibiotics alone can be given. Antibiotics to combat skin organisms, such as *Staphylococci*, and gut bacteria including anaerobes are routinely given after the drainage procedure.

Anal fistula
Clinical features
Anal fistula is usually manifest as intermittent discharge over the perianal area from the fistula. The fistula itself can be seen as a small area of granulation tissue around the anal margin. It is often dismissed as incomplete healing of anorectal abscesses. Underlying Crohn's disease should be excluded or confirmed.

Diagnosis and evaluation
Examination performed with the patient under anesthesia is usually required to establish the site of the proximal opening by a probe. Occasionally, a dye is injected into the distal orifice to identify the opening (fistulogram).

Etiology and pathogenesis
Anal fistula is a common complication of anorectal abscesses as the anal gland infection spreads to form an abscess and drains externally in the form of a fistula. Magnetic resonance imaging demonstrating an anal fistula is shown in Fig. 17.15. Crohn's disease is also a cause of anal fistulas, and they are often multiple.

Treatment
Once the proximal opening has been identified, the fistula can be laid open and healing by secondary intention occurs, provided the fistula does not involve the anal sphincter.

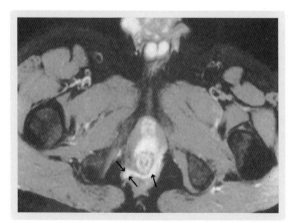

Fig. 17.15 Magnetic resonance scan demonstration of anal fistula tracking around the back of the anal canal and through the muscularis on the right side (arrows).

Fistulas that involve the sphincter will require a specialist anorectal surgeon for preservation and repair of the sphincter to ensure continence.

Fistulas caused by Crohn's disease should be treated with conservative treatment, as for active Crohn's disease. Surgical treatment usually involves an ileostomy.

Infections

Bacterial infection of the colon
Incidence
Bacterial infection of the colon is the most common cause of diarrhea worldwide, especially afflicting travelers outside their own country.

Clinical features
Typical symptoms of bacterial infection of the colon include:
- Diarrhea, abdominal pain, fever, and vomiting.
- Leukocytosis, seen on full blood count.

Clinical and biochemical evidence of dehydration is not uncommon, especially at extreme of ages (i.e., in elderly persons and infants).

Diagnosis and evaluation
Tests of use include:
- Routine biochemistry and complete blood count.
- Stool culture.
- Sigmoidoscopy and biopsy, if diarrhea is persistent.

Etiology and pathogenesis
Common pathogens include species of *Escherichia coli*, *Shigella*, and *Salmonella*, which are spread via the fecal-oral route and are often the result of poor food hygiene. Invasion of the colonic epithelium occurs, and in some cases with certain strains of *E. coli*, an enterotoxin is produced.

Clostridium difficile infection is typically seen after broad-spectrum antibiotic therapy, especially when clindamycin is involved. Disturbance of normal colonic flora caused by antibiotics allows proliferation of C. *difficile* and toxin production. On sigmoidoscopy, plaques of inflammatory exudates can be seen, giving the appearance of pseudomembranes (i.e., pseudomembranous colitis). Direct person-to-person spread can also occur.

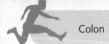

Diagnosis can be made by isolation of the toxins in the stool.

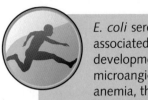

E. coli serotype 0157 is associated with the development of a microangiopathic hemolytic anemia, thrombocytopenia, and renal failure, often requiring dialysis. This is termed "hemolytic uremic syndrome" (HUS) and has an associated mortality rate.

Treatment

Adequate rehydration and electrolyte correction are required either intravenously or orally.

Once stool cultures have confirmed the diagnosis, appropriate antibiotics should be started. If the patient is severely ill, ciprofloxacin can be started empirically once stool and blood culture samples have been taken. If C. *difficile* is suspected or confirmed, oral metronidazole or vancomycin is the drug of choice.

Antidiarrheal agents such as codeine or loperamide should be avoided if possible because they impair the clearance of the pathogen from the bowel.

Amebiasis
Incidence
Amebiasis occurs worldwide but more commonly in the tropics.

Clinical features
In acute infection, typical symptoms include:
- Abdominal pain.
- Diarrhea (often bloody).
- Nausea and vomiting.

Fulminant colitis and toxic dilatation can occur, though rarely.

Diagnosis and evaluation
Useful tests in determining the diagnosis include the following:
- Fresh stool samples are required for the identification of amebic cysts.
- Specific antibodies can be measured in the serum.
- Sigmoidoscopy demonstrates ulceration of the colonic mucosa, but it is not diagnostic.

Etiology and pathogenesis
Amebiasis is caused by *Entamoeba histolytica*, which is digested in its cyst form via contaminated food or water or direct person-to-person spread. Multiplication of the organisms takes place in the colon, where they invade the colonic epithelium and cause ulceration. Not all who are infected will have clinical disease, and some become asymptomatic cyst carriers.

Complications
Complications of amebiasis are uncommon. Perforation due to toxic dilatation can occur, and strictures can occur in chronic infection.

Hepatic abscesses are not uncommon (see Chapter 18).

Treatment
Metronidazole is the drug of choice for the treatment of amebiasis. Education and advice regarding hygiene can help reduce person-to-person spread.

Cryptosporidiosis
Clinical features
Symptoms include:
- Watery diarrhea.
- Fever.
- Abdominal pain.

Toxic dilatation and a sclerosing cholangitis-like picture can be seen in patients with AIDS.

Diagnosis and evaluation
Parasites can be identified by modified Ziehl-Neelsen stain of feces or intestinal biopsy. Fecal oocysts should be quantified.

Etiology and pathogenesis
The fungal parasite is found worldwide, with its major reservoir in cattle, and is likely to be spread via contaminated water supplies.

Healthy persons will have a self-limiting gastroenteritis, and often the diagnosis is not confirmed. Persons who are immunocompromised tend to have a devastating illness with protracted episodes of diarrhea.

The infective organism also causes sclerosing cholangitis in immunocompromised patients.

Treatment
Cryptosporidiosis may be self-limiting if the CD4 lymphocyte count is not too suppressed.

Paromomycin has been shown to be effective. Good hygiene prevents spread of the infection.

Schistosomiasis

See also Chapter 18.

Clinical features

The main features of schistosomiasis are:

- Fever.
- Urticaria.
- Nausea.
- Vomiting.
- Bloody diarrhea.

Diagnosis and evaluation

Consider the following tests:

- Specific antibodies can be detected by serology.
- Eggs can be isolated from stool, urine, or rectal biopsy.
- Sigmoidoscopy reveals mucosal ulceration, which as an isolated finding, is not diagnostic.

Etiology and pathogenesis

Schistosoma mansoni predominantly affects the colon, causing erythema and ulceration of the mucosa. A localized granulomatous reaction may be mistaken for colonic cancer. Progressive fibrosis leads to stricture formation, but obstruction is rare.

S. japonicum affects the small intestine and proximal colon, and epithelial dysplasia is seen with chronic infection, which is now accepted to be a premalignant condition.

Complications

Periportal fibrosis and portal hypertension can ensue. Another possible complication is ectopic deposition of eggs elsewhere in the body (e.g., lung and brain).

Treatment

The drug of choice is praziquantel because it is effective against all human schistosomes, combining broad-spectrum activity with low toxicity.

Whipworm infection

Incidence

Whipworm infection occurs worldwide. The prevalence can be as high as 90% in economically poor communities with poor hygiene.

Clinical features

Whipworm infection is usually asymptomatic.

Heavy infestation causes bloody diarrhea associated with weight loss, abdominal discomfort, and anorexia. Involvement of the appendix causes appendicitis.

Diagnosis and evaluation

Stool examination for eggs is the recommended test.

With sigmoidoscopy, adult worms may be seen attached to the rectal mucosa.

Etiology and pathogenesis

Whipworm infection is caused by *Trichuris trichiura*. Adult worms are more commonly found in the distal ileum and cecum. The whole colon may be affected in heavy infection.

The adult worm embeds itself in the colonic mucosa, causing damage and ulceration and leading to protein and blood loss in severe cases.

Treatment

The anthelmintic mebendazole is the treatment of choice, but its use needs to be combined with hygienic measures to break the cycle of autoinfection. All family members should receive therapy.

Threadworm infection

Incidence

Threadworm infection occurs worldwide but is more prevalent in temperate climates. Outbreaks are seen in institutional establishments and areas of overcrowded living conditions.

Clinical features

Pruritus ani is intense and usually nocturnal due to egg laying by the female threadworm.

Submucosal abscess is rare and due to secondary bacterial infection of the colonic mucosa.

Diagnosis and evaluation

Adult worms may be seen directly leaving the anus. Clear adhesive tape can be applied to the perianal region to allow for the identification of eggs microscopically.

Etiology and pathogenesis

Threadworm infection is caused by *Enterobius vermicularis* and commonly affects children. Adult worms reside in the colon, and female worms migrate to the perianal region to lay their eggs. Superficial

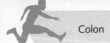

damage to the colonic mucosa is common during heavy infestations.

Autoinfection via scratching and poor hygiene aggravates the problem. Rarely, migration to the peritoneum and visceral organs occurs.

Treatment

Mebendazole given as two single doses, 2 weeks apart, is effective in treating threadworm infection. Asymptomatic family members should also be treated.

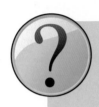

- What drugs can be implicated in causing constipation?
- What are the contrasting features between ulcerative colitis and Crohn's disease?
- What are the clinical and laboratory features that indicate a severe exacerbation of ulcerative colitis?
- How would you manage a patient presenting with an acute severe exacerbation of ulcerative colitis?
- What are the potential indications for surgery in ulcerative colitis?
- What is Dukes' classification of colonic cancer?
- What is the pathophysiology of *Clostridium difficile* infection? Which antibiotics in particular are implicated?

18. Liver

Structure and function of the liver

The predominant pathologic mechanisms affecting the liver are:
- Necrosis.
- Inflammation.
- Fibrosis.

The site at which these disease processes occur may produce different clinical syndromes, and the functions of the liver (Fig. 18.1) may be affected differentially:
- Centrilobular processes affect synthetic and metabolic functions, and hepatocellular necrosis produces an enzyme rise predominantly of alanine transaminase (ALT) and aspartate transaminase (AST) (Fig. 18.2).
- Centrifugal or periportal processes have less effect on synthetic function but disproportionate effects on portal pressure and bile duct excretory function. Disease here tends to cause disproportionate increase in the "biliary" enzymes alkaline phosphatase and gamma glutamyl transferase (see Fig. 18.2).
- Alcoholic liver disease tends to have effects throughout all parts of the lobule, and most

Functions of the liver	
Function	**Substrate examples**
Synthetic function	Albumin (half-life 20 days) Transferrin (half-life 3 days) Coagulation factors (all of them)
Storage	Glycogen, triglyceride, iron (ferritin), vitamin A
Metabolic homeostasis	Maintenance blood glucose (glycogenolysis and gluconeogenesis)
Metabolic activation and transformation	Vitamin D, lipoproteins
Metabolic deactivation and detoxification	Sex steroids, ammonia, drugs, alcohol
Excretion	Bilirubin

Fig. 18.1 Functions of the liver.

progressive diseases ultimately will also involve both portal tracts and centrilobular areas.

Hyperbilirubinemias

Unconjugated hyperbilirubinemia
Gilbert's syndrome
Incidence and diagnosis
Gilbert's syndrome is the most common congenital hyperbilirubinemia, affecting 2–5% of the population. It is:
- Usually detected incidentally on routine checks as an isolated, raised bilirubin level.
- More commonly manifest in males.

The patient is often asymptomatic, and a positive family history of jaundice may be seen in 5–10% of cases. Serum bilirubin is usually less than 3 mg/dL (normal level, <1.2 mg/dL). Intercurrent illness such as infection tends to elevate bilirubin levels.

Diagnosis can be made on the basis of an increase in unconjugated bilirubin following an overnight fast or during a mild illness. A genetic test is now available to confirm TATA box elongation in Gilbert's syndrome (see below).

Etiology and pathogenesis
Etiology of Gilbert's syndrome involves a reduction in enzyme activity (UDP-glucuronosyl-transferase [UGT–1]), but many other factors can affect this—hence its variable presentation. UGT–1 is a cytoplasmic enzyme that conjugates bilirubin to allow it to be excreted in a soluble form. Recently, a mutation in the promoter region (TATA box) of the messenger RNA for this enzyme was described, which reduces the efficiency of transcription of this enzyme. The normal enzyme is present but is less efficient due to reduced synthesis. It is possible that Gilbert's syndrome represents an extreme end of a normal distribution.

Prognosis
Gilbert's syndrome carries an excellent prognosis. It is important to reassure the patient that the condition is not serious and avoid any unnecessary evaluations in the future. No treatment is required.

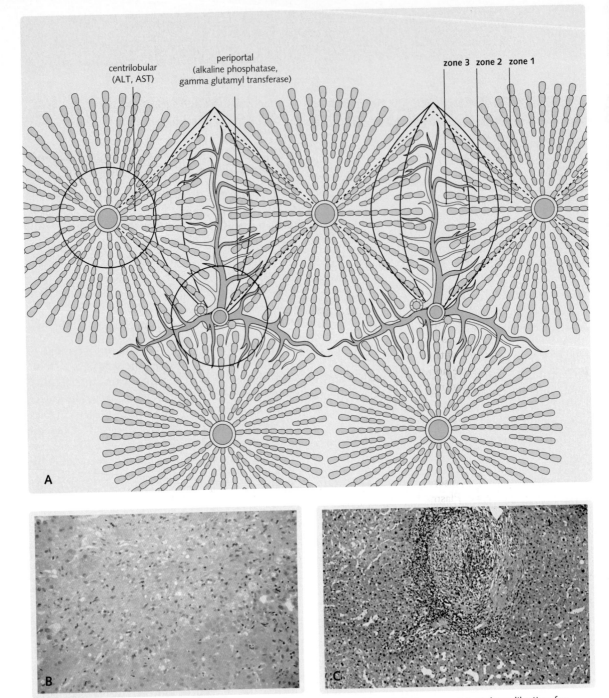

Fig. 18.2 A. Hepatic lobular architecture showing functional zones and centrilobular or centripetal predilection for pathologic processes. Different enzymes predominate in the different zones, and their detection in serum may reflect liver damage in those zones. B. Centrilobular necrosis with inflammation. C. Inflammation centered on portal tract with early fibrosis.

Crigler-Najjar syndrome

Crigler-Najjar syndrome is a more severe unconjugated hyperbilirubinemia, again due to abnormalities of the UGT–1 enzyme (same as in Gilbert's syndrome). Here, the mutations are in the translated region of DNA, not just the promoter region, so the enzyme may not be produced at all. Two types have been described, both of which are exceedingly rare conditions:

- Type I (autosomal recessive)—complete absence of glucuronosyltransferase.
- Type II (autosomal dominant)—decreased level of glucuronosyltransferase.

Type I deficiency presents as neonatal jaundice due to unconjugated bilirubinemia and is usually fatal within the first year of life. Serum bilirubin levels can rise to 30 to 50 mg/dL. Death occurs from kernicterus, possibly due to an immature blood-brain barrier.

Type II deficiency survival into adulthood is not uncommon. The serum bilirubin level is usually less than 20 mg/dL. Kernicterus can be prevented by induction of the enzyme with phenobarbitone.

Liver biopsy results are normal, and transplantation is the only treatment for debilitated patients.

Conjugated hyperbilirubinemia
Dubin-Johnson syndrome
Incidence and diagnosis

This is a rare and benign disorder that usually presents in adolescence. Plasma bilirubin is conjugated.

A Bromosulfthalein clearance test in Dubin-Johnson syndrome has a second recirculation peak at 90 minutes (see Chapter 24, Liver enzymes and liver function tests). The liver biopsy specimen is stained black due to centrilobular melanin deposits.

Etiology and pathogenesis

Dubin-Johnson syndrome is believed to result from failure to excrete conjugated bilirubin due to a defect in a transporter protein in the bile canaliculi. The inheritance is autosomal recessive.

Prognosis and treatment

No specific treatment is required, and the prognosis is excellent.

Rotor syndrome

Rotor syndrome is a benign and probably autosomal dominant condition of conjugated hyperbilirubinemia. It can be distinguished from Dubin-Johnson syndrome by a normal liver biopsy. Prognosis is also excellent for this syndrome.

Viral hepatitis

Traditionally, viruses with a predilection to cause hepatitis have come to be classified alphabetically. Currently, at least six different viruses are known to infect humans (A, B, C, D, E, and G). Other viruses such as cytomegalovirus (CMV), Epstein-Barr virus (EBV), yellow fever virus, and herpesvirus can also infect the liver.

Hepatitis A
Incidence

Hepatitis A is the most common type of hepatitis worldwide, with young persons most frequently afflicted. Epidemics are associated with overcrowding, poor hygiene, and poor sanitation. Transmission occurs by the fecal-oral route or through the ingestion of contaminated water or shellfish.

Clinical features

In the prodromal phase:
- Symptoms mimic viral gastroenteritis (e.g., nausea, vomiting, diarrhea, headache, mild fever, malaise, and abdominal discomfort).
- A distaste for cigarettes is said to be characteristic in young adults who normally smoke them.

The icteric phase occurs after 10 to 14 days (some patients remain anicteric) and resolves in 2 to 3 weeks:
- Mild symptoms such as malaise and fatigue may persist for months.
- Liver enlargement is common during the icteric phase; the spleen is palpable in approximately 10% of cases.

Diagnosis and evaluation

Diagnosis is usually made on clinical grounds. A definitive diagnosis can be made if there is a rising titer of anti–hepatitis A virus (HAV) immunoglobulin (Ig) M and/or demonstration of viral particles in stools by electron microscopy. An elevated anti-HAV IgG titer reflects previous exposure to hepatitis A and thus lifelong immunity.

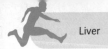

Transaminases are moderately elevated (500 to 1000 IU/L) but normalize rapidly (Fig. 18.3).

Etiology and pathogenesis
Hepatitis A is a pico-RNA-virus excreted in the feces of an infected person approximately 2 weeks before the onset of jaundice and up to 1 week thereafter. The disease is most infectious just before the onset of jaundice. The RNA virus is relatively heat resistant, withstanding 60°C for up to 30 minutes; hence, it thrives in areas of poor hygiene.

Complications
Complications are rare in cases of hepatitis A, but myocarditis, arthritis, vasculitis, and occasionally fulminant hepatic failure have been described.

Prognosis
Most patients recover completely without any sequelae; some have a self-limiting relapse of hepatitis. A few have a prolonged cholestatic jaundice (3 to 4 months), but in general the prognosis is excellent. Often, the course is more prolonged in adults or immunocompromised patients.

Hepatitis A infection does not have a carrier status. Progression to chronic viral disease does not occur but in some persons may precipitate autoimmune liver disease. Previous infection confers lifetime immunity.

Aims and indication for treatment
Unless a patient infected with hepatitis A is very unwell, hospital admission is unnecessary. Treatment otherwise is supportive.

Vaccination or hyperimmune globulin should be offered to persons at high risk.

Treatment
Antiemetic agents can be given for nausea and vomiting, intravenous fluids for dehydration, and simple analgesia for headaches. It is important to maintain caloric intake. Alcohol should be avoided.

Hepatitis B
Incidence
The rate of infected carriers of hepatitis B not exhibiting symptoms is 0.1% in the United States and the United Kingdom and 20% in parts of Asia and Africa. The worldwide prevalence of carriers is estimated at 300 to 400 million persons.

Transmission takes place via the following routes:
- Contaminated blood products. Incidence has fallen dramatically since the introduction of screening in the United States and Europe in the late 1970s and, subsequently, around the world with the World Health Organization vaccination program.
- Contaminated needles (common among intravenous drug users [IVDUs]).
- Sexual intercourse with an infected partner.
- Vertical transmission (most common mode worldwide).
- Viral particles have been isolated from insects such as mosquitoes, but whether mosquitoes can transmit the disease remains unproven.

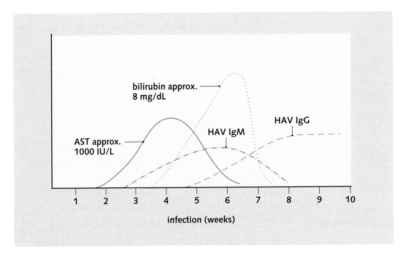

Fig. 18.3 Laboratory tests and their time course in hepatitis A infection.

Etiology and pathogenesis

Hepatitis B virus (HBV) is a DNA virus that replicates in the liver where the core antigen incorporates itself into the host genome. The host's DNA polymerase then transcribes for the virus and may be the prime factor for the development of hepatocellular carcinoma. HBV has 3200 base nucleotides with four open reading frames that encode for surface antigens (pS1, pS2, S), core antigens (pre-core and core antigen), DNA polymerase, and X proteins. X proteins are thought to play an important role in carcinogenesis. Mutation at the pre-core and core-promoter region leads to "pre-core mutants" that do not express hepatitis B e antigen (HBeAg) in the serum despite active replication. It is important to understand that the pre-core mutant type of HBV infection has become increasingly common in the United States and is widely prevalent in Asia and Mediterranean countries.

Body fluid contact is essential for transmission. Infection in the birth canal during parturition is the most important mode worldwide, creating a large "carrier state" reservoir of infection. In developed countries, those who engage in promiscuous sex and IVDUs form the largest reservoir of infection.

Hepatitis B syndromes may be acute, chronic, or in the carrier state.

Clinical features

Features of acute hepatitis B include the following:
- The incubation time is 60 to 160 days (average, 90 days).
- Nonspecific prodromal symptoms include arthralgia, anorexia, and abdominal discomfort.
- Jaundice, fever, and hepatomegaly are usual features.
- Urticarial or maculopapular rash may appear, together with a polyarthritis thought to be secondary to immune-mediated complexes.
- A history of contact with a contaminated source is usual (especially travelers to the Orient, drug addicts, accidental injury to health workers, etc.).

Features of chronic hepatitis B include the following:
- Most chronic carriers are asymptomatic.
- The majority of cases are discovered incidentally (e.g., blood donor screening, occupational health checks, routine liver function tests).
- Patients with chronic active hepatitis may present with features or complications of chronic liver disease, or cirrhosis: jaundice, ascites, portal hypertension, hepatic failure.

- Chronic hepatitis predisposes to cirrhosis of the liver and an increased risk of hepatocellular carcinoma, especially in men.

Diagnosis and evaluation

Transaminase levels may be very high in the acute stage (1000 to 5000 IU/L), falling rapidly after the first week; chronic hepatitis produces only a mild elevation of ALT or AST.

Serologic tests are summarized in Fig. 18.4. Surface antigen (HBsAg) is the first serologic marker to appear (6 weeks to 3 months). HBeAg follows, reflecting viral replication, high infectivity, and more severe disease. It usually disappears before HBsAg, but its persistence correlates with HBV DNA in blood. HBsAg and HBeAg may be present in either acute or chronic HBV infection.

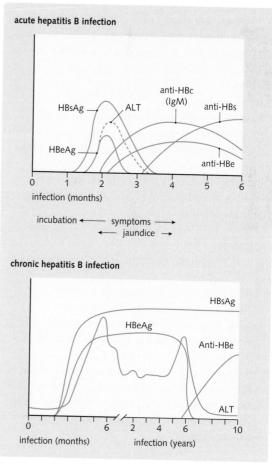

Fig. 18.4 Laboratory tests and their time course in hepatitis B infection. (Redrawn from Kumar PJ, Clarke ML: *Clinical Medicine,* 3rd ed. London, Baillière Tindall, 1994.)

Anti-HBe antibodies appear from approximately 8 weeks after infection, and their presence reflects low infectivity. Such seroconversion may occur spontaneously after several decades or with interferon. Anti-HBs antibodies appear late (>3 months) and confer lifelong immunity.

Antibodies to the core antigen (HBcAg, IgM) were measured in the past when there was a window period during which HBsAg disappeared and anti-HBsAg was not detectable, but this has been largely superseded by detection of core DNA by polymerase chain reaction (PCR).

It is important to understand the differences in serology between "wild" type and "pre-core mutant" type HBV infection (Fig. 18.5). In wild type, in the presence of active replication (high HBV DNA), HBeAg will be positive and hepatitis B e antibody (HBeAb) will be negative. In the pre-core mutant type, HBeAg will be negative, and HBeAb will be positive, even in the presence of active replication (high HBV DNA). This important distinction is critical to assess active HBV infection and to understand the role of treatment.

Complications

Fulminant hepatitis and death occur in 1% of patients. Extrahepatic complications such as arteritis and glomerulonephritis may be immune-complex mediated. Cryoglobulinemia may also occur. Variations in the viral genome (mutants) are becoming more common, often associated with fulminant hepatitis.

Prognosis

Up to 90% of acute hepatitis B infections resolve without sequelae:

- Five to ten percent of patients become chronic carriers. The carrier rate is much higher after vertical transmission, possibly due to immature immune response to the virus in the neonate.
- Five percent develop chronic active hepatitis, which may progress to cirrhosis or hepatocellular carcinoma in cirrhotic patients, especially males (25% lifetime risk for hepatocellular carcinoma in cirrhotic males).

Aims of treatment

For acute hepatitis B infection, as in hepatitis A infection, symptomatic relief is all that is required,

Serology of wild type and pre-core mutant HBV infection		
Test	HBeAg-positive (wild type)	HBeAg-negative (pre-core mutant)
HBsAg	Positive	Positive
HBeAg	Positive	Negative
HBeAb	Negative	Positive
HBV DNA	High	High
AST/ALT	May be elevated	May be elevated
Histology	May show chronic hepatitis or cirrhosis	May show chronic hepatitis or cirrhosis

Fig. 18.5 Serology of wild-type and pre-core mutant type HBV infection.

with extra precautions taken when handling body fluids. Fulminant hepatitis carries a grave prognosis and requires intensive care and potentially liver transplantation. Chronic hepatitis B is treated only in the presence of active inflammation, fibrosis, or cirrhosis. There is no evidence to suggest that treatment will be beneficial or successful in "inactive carriers." Inactive carriers will have active replication but persistently normal AST/ALT and normal liver histology. When treating chronic HBV infection, the aims of treatments are different for wild and pre-core mutant types of HBV.

In wild-type HBV, the goal of treatment is seroconversion. However, in pre-core mutant HBV, patients may need to be treated lifelong or until HBsAg disappears (Fig. 18.6).

Currently, there are a number of treatment options for patients with chronic HBV infection (Fig. 18.7). Although some of these drugs are used as monotherapy, in the future many of these drugs may be used in combination to reduce the risk of drug-resistant mutations.

Vaccination is successful in preventing transmission. When combined with immunoglobulin at birth, this successfully prevents vertical transmission. Hyperimmune globulin and/or lamivudine, nucleoside reverse transcriptase inhibitors, are used to prevent recurrence after transplantation.

Indication for treatment

Patients who have evidence of active replication (high HBV DNA) and evidence of chronic hepatitis

Goals of treatment in HBV infection	
Wild type (HBeAg-positive)	Pre-core mutant (HBeAg-negative)
Seroconversion is the main goal	Seroconversion is not the goal since HBeAg is negative and HBeAb is positive before treatment
HBeAg-positive → HBeAg-negative	Treatment is lifelong or until HBsAg disappears
HBeAb-negative → HBeAb-positive	High relapse rates if treatment is discontinued
Durability of response after seroconversion 80%	Treatment response can be monitored by HBV DNA levels

Fig. 18.6 Goals of treatment in HBV infection.

Treatment options for HBV infection	
Drug	Comments
Interferon alpha	Contraindicated in decompensated liver disease Short duration of treatment (~ 4 months)
Lamivudine (Epivir)	Orally administered nucleoside analog Drug resistance due to mutations with prolonged treatment (up to 70% after 5 years)
Adefovir dipivoxil (Hepsera)	Orally administered nucleoside analog Durg resistance in up to 18% after 3 years
Entecavir (Baraclude)	Oral nucleoside analog Only early experience, but drug resistance may be a problem
Tenofovir (Viread)	Not approved for treatment of HBV by FDA Limited experience, but effective
Combination treatment	Trials are in progress to improve efficacy and reduce drug resistance

Fig. 18.7 Treatment options for HBV infection.

or cirrhosis on liver histology should be considered for treatment (Fig. 18.8).

Treatment plan

Subcutaneous injection of interferon alpha or pegylated interferon can induce seroconversion in 33–40% of cases. Interferon is more effective in patients with high inflammatory activity on liver biopsy and low viral loads. It is contraindicated in decompensated cirrhosis and should be used with extreme caution in the presence of cirrhosis since patients may decompensate on treatment. Significant side effects, including fatigue, arthralgia, pyrexia, depression, and neutropenia, limit the tolerability of the drug.

The nucleoside/nucleotide analogs, including lamivudine, adefovir, and entecavir, offer much better safety profiles. Seroconversion in HBeAg-positive (wild-type HBV) patients ranges from 15–20% after 1 year of treatment, with higher seroconversion with prolonged treatment. These drugs are very well tolerated with minimal side effects, but drug resistance is a major problem, especially with lamivudine. Lamivudine resistance (YMDD mutation) develops at the rate of 17–20% per year of treatment. Lamivudine-resistant strains are often sensitive to adefovir or entecavir. Adefovir is a nucleotide analog with an excellent safety profile and relatively low drug resistance. There are ongoing trials using these drugs with or without interferon in an effort to reduce drug resistance and improve efficacy.

All patients with chronic hepatitis B should be vaccinated against hepatitis A, and their family members should be screened and vaccinated for hepatitis B.

All pregnant women positive for HBV should plan for vaccination of the newborn at parturition. Vaccination should also be offered to other persons at risk, such as IVDUs, health care personnel, and travelers to high-risk areas.

Poor prognostic factors in hepatitis B and C	
Hepatitis B	**Hepatitis C**
Possibly duration of infection; age >40 years	Age at acquisition: older fare worse
Any signs (e.g., spider nevi, ascites)	Presence of decompensation, such as ascites, encephalopathy, or variceal bleeding
Activity on liver biopsy, especially if cirrhotic	Bridging fibrosis or cirrhosis on liver biopsy
Males fare worse than females	Males fare worse than females
Concomitant disease	Possibly higher iron stores and alcohol intake cause synergistic damage
Development of hepatocellular carcinoma, especially in males	Development of hepatocellular carcinoma, especially in males

Fig. 18.8 Poor prognostic factors in hepatitis B and C.

Hepatitis C
Incidence
Previously known as "non-A, non-B hepatitis," hepatitis C is now thought to be responsible for up to 90% of such cases. The hepatitis C virus (HCV) was identified in 1988, and routine screening of blood products has been available only since 1991.

Transmission occurs via:
- Contaminated blood products.
- Contaminated instrumentation (such as needles used by IVDUs).
- Sexual, vertical, or breast milk transmission is uncommon (less than 5%).

Clinical features
Features of hepatitis C include the following:
- Clinical jaundice occurs in less than 20% of patients.
- Sixty-five to seventy percent of those infected develop chronic hepatitis and 20% develop cirrhosis; 5% (15% with cirrhosis) develop hepatocellular carcinoma (HCC) during their lifetime.
- Fatigue and malaise are common.
- Extrahepatic manifestations such as arthritis, cryoglobulinemia, and aplastic anemia are rare.

A minority of patients with cirrhosis may have its attendant potential complications of portal hypertension, hepatic failure, or hepatoma.

Diagnosis
Most commonly, patients are referred for investigation of abnormal liver enzymes found incidentally or are referred by the blood transfusion service when they are discovered to be antibody positive.
- Transaminase levels are usually only slightly elevated (ALT, 50 to 150 IU/L).
- Bilirubin and synthetic function test results are usually normal.
- Antibodies to hepatitis C are found in the serum using enzyme-linked immunosorbent assay or radioimmunoassay kits.
- Viral RNA is detectable by reverse transcriptase–PCR (RT-PCR); a positive result confirms current viremia.
- Viral genotyping is important before treatment because the duration of and the response to treatment are dependent on genotype. Genotype 1 is common in the United States, composing 70–80% of all infection. Genotypes 2 and 3 are less common, composing 20–30%, whereas genotypes 4, 5, and 6 are found in other parts of the world.
- Liver histology can demonstrate a spectrum of change, from fatty infiltration through lobular hepatitis to cirrhosis. These changes correlate poorly to liver enzyme derangement.

Etiology and pathogenesis
Hepatitis C is a single-stranded RNA virus with several immunogenic subtypes that could be used in epidemiologic studies to establish modes of transmission.

Complications and prognosis
The complications and prognosis of hepatitis C are as follows:
- Seventy percent of patients contract chronic indolent hepatitis of varying severity.
- Twenty percent of cases progress to cirrhosis.

Advanced age, male sex, alcoholism, and fibrosis on liver biopsy are independent factors that predict progression to cirrhosis (see Fig. 18.8). Progression is also much more rapid in the presence of coinfection with HIV. Fulminant hepatitis is a rare but fatal complication.

Aims of treatment
The main aim of treatment is to eradicate the virus (i.e., sustained viral clearance or sustained virologic

response [SVR]). Clearance of the virus leads to improvement in liver histology and prevents disease progression.

The end point of treatment is the achievement of SVR, that is, undetectable virus in the serum as tested by sensitive PCR technique at 6 months after completion of treatment. Patients who achieve SVR have been shown to have extremely low relapse rates (<2%).

Indications for treatment

All patients with hepatitis C who have significant inflammation or fibrosis should be considered for treatment. The treatment of patients with persistently normal liver enzyme levels is controversial and probably not indicated unless there is evidence of inflammation or fibrosis on liver biopsy.

Low viral counts, genotypes 2 and 3, absence of significant fibrosis or cirrhosis, young age, and white race predict higher SVR rates.

Treatment plan

Patients with hepatitis C should be counseled regarding modes of transmission and advised against excess alcohol consumption, which appears to accelerate progression of the disease.

Interferon is rarely used as monotherapy for the treatment of HCV except in those persons who cannot tolerate ribavirin because of side effects or renal failure. Combination treatment with pegylated interferon and ribavirin is currently considered the standard treatment. Pegylation (i.e., attaching a molecule of polyethylene glycol to interferon alpha) increases the half-life by decreasing renal clearance and improves efficacy. Pegylated interferon is administered once a week in combination with weight-based ribavirin (nucleoside analog) daily in divided doses. Patients with genotypes 2 and 3 are treated for 24 weeks and those with other genotypes are treated for 48 weeks. If there is no response to treatment (i.e., negative HCV RNA by PCR or 2-log reduction in viral load) at 12 weeks, treatment may be discontinued because continued treatment is unlikely to be beneficial.

Response rates vary by viral load, genotype, age, sex, and severity of fibrosis on liver biopsy (bridging fibrosis or cirrhosis). In general, high viral load (>2 million IU/mL), genotype 1, male sex, age older than 50 years, immunosuppression, and the presence of cirrhosis are poor prognostic factors predicting low

SVR rates. Genotypes 2 and 3 are highly responsive to treatment, with SVR rates of 80–90% after 6 months of therapy, whereas genotype 1 requires a year of treatment with SVR rates of 45–55%. Patients should be monitored carefully for side effects of therapy, which include suicidal ideation, visual changes, weight loss, hypothyroidism or hyperthyroidism, and depression of hematologic parameters including anemia, leukopenia, and thrombocytopenia.

Patients with hepatitis C should be vaccinated against hepatitis A and B if they do not have native immunity. Centers for Disease Control and Prevention guidelines do not recommend changing sexual practices among monogamous partners as a means of prevention due to the low risk of sexual transmission.

Hepatitis D
Incidence

Also known as the delta virus, hepatitis D is an incomplete RNA particle that is unable to replicate by itself. It occurs as a coinfection with HBV and is particularly seen in IVDUs, but it can affect any patient with hepatitis B.

Diagnosis

The coinfection of hepatitis B and D is indistinguishable from acute hepatitis B infection, but occasionally superinfection produces an active flare-up of hepatitis with a rise of liver transaminases. Clinical jaundice may not be obvious.

The presence of IgM antidelta virus with IgM anti-HBcAg confirms coinfection, and IgM anti-delta is replaced by IgG antidelta over 6 to 8 weeks. IgM antidelta in the presence of IgG anti-HBcAg indicates superinfection because IgM anti-HBcAg is replaced by IgG antibodies after the initial infection. Hepatitis D RNA can be measured in the serum and liver and is seen in both acute and chronic infection.

Etiology and pathogenesis

The incomplete RNA particle is enclosed within HBsAg, suggesting that it is unable to replicate by itself but is activated in the presence of hepatitis B infection.

Complications

Fulminant hepatitis is a serious complication and is more common after coinfection. Chronic infection with hepatitis D usually causes cirrhosis.

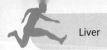

Aims of treatment

Treatment is supportive for fulminant hepatitis. Reduction of viral replication with interferon to reduce the risk of developing cirrhosis is also recommended for chronic infection.

Indications for treatment

Chronic active hepatitis as demonstrated on liver enzyme tests and biopsy is indicative of treatment.

Treatment plan

The treatment plan for hepatitis D should proceed as it would for other types of chronic viral hepatitis with interferon alpha, which can induce remission; however, as with hepatitis C infection, relapse is common on withdrawal of treatment.

Hepatitis E

In summary:

- Hepatitis E is an RNA virus spread via the fecal-oral route.
- Infection with hepatitis E is predominantly seen in developing countries.
- Mortality rises from 1–20% in pregnant women; the reason is at present unclear.
- Hepatitis E RNA can be detected in serum or stool by PCR.
- Treatment, as for hepatitis A, is purely symptomatic.
- There is no carrier state and no progression to chronic active hepatitis.
- Improved sanitation and hygiene are essential for prevention and control.

A summary of hepatitis viruses is shown in Fig. 18.9.

Hepatitis G

Hepatitis G (also called GB-C) has recently been identified and has some sequence homology with hepatitis C. It has been found in about 2% of blood donors who have been screened, but there is no routine screening test available. It is thought not to cause acute or chronic hepatitis, and its precise clinical relevance is still not clear.

Epstein-Barr virus (infectious mononucleosis)

Incidence and diagnosis

EBV infection is a common disease of the young, although it can occur at any age.

Fever, malaise, and tonsillar and glandular enlargement are typical; mild jaundice associated with abnormal liver function tests is common. Rash can occur, particularly if the patient is given ampicillin (this does not imply future ampicillin allergy).

Heterophile antibodies (Paul-Bunnell or Monospot) can be detected early and disappear after 3 months. They agglutinate sheep red blood cells but do not react with EBV or its antigens. False-positive Monospot test results can occasionally occur in other viral illness, lymphomas, or systemic lupus erythematosus. An increase in IgM antibodies specific to EBV is diagnostic of infectious mononucleosis. In addition, atypical, reactive lymphocytes can be seen on a peripheral blood film.

Etiology and pathogenesis

Usually transmitted via saliva (infectious mononucleosis is also known as "kissing disease"), EBV infection has an incubation time of 4 to 5 weeks.

Hepatitis viruses				
Type	Spread	Incubation	Prevention	Treatment
A	Fecal-oral	2–6 weeks	Immunoglobulin or vaccine	Not specific
B	Contaminated body fluid: vertical, blood, semen	2–6 months	Hepatitis B immunoglobulin or vaccine	Interferon alpha Lamivudine, adefovir, entecavir
C	Contaminated blood	6–8 weeks	None available	Interferon alpha Ribavirin
D	Contaminated blood Requires hepatitis B	Unknown	Prevention of hepatitis B	None
E	Fecal-oral	2–9 weeks	Improve hygiene	None

Fig. 18.9 Summary of hepatitis viruses.

Large mononuclear cells are seen to infiltrate the portal tracts, but liver architecture is preserved.

Complications and prognosis

Hepatitis due to EBV carries an excellent prognosis, with a majority of patients retaining normal liver function. Splenomegaly and hemolytic anemia can also occur.

Cytomegalovirus

Cytomegalovirus infection occurs predominantly in immunosuppressed patients, occasionally causing a hepatitis with fatal consequences.

- CMV may be detected in urine, but isolation and growth are slow.
- The most sensitive test is to detect CMV antigen in buffy coat of ethylenediaminetetraacetic acid peripheral blood. PCR technology can also be used.
- A rising IgM titer to CMV can also be seen to aid diagnosis of acute infection.
- Liver biopsy reveals intracytoplasmic inclusion bodies and giant cells.

Other infections involving the liver

Toxoplasmosis

Toxoplasmosis is rare in the United States. Clinical features in an adult are often indistinguishable from infectious mononucleosis caused by EBV (negative Monospot test).

A congenital form of the infection can occur if a mother is infected during pregnancy.

Clinical features

Most toxoplasmosis infections are asymptomatic. Lymphadenopathy associated with a febrile illness is the most common form of presentation.

Maculopapular rash, hepatosplenomegaly, and reactive lymphocytes may be seen together with a biochemical rise in serum transaminase levels with or without clinical hepatitis. Rarely, chorioretinitis, myocarditis, or encephalitis can occur, but this is more commonly observed in immunocompromised persons.

Diagnosis

Rising IgM titers are diagnostic (although unreliable in HIV-positive patients). The infective organism can also be isolated by injecting tissues (e.g., bone marrow or cerebrospinal fluid from the patient) into the peritoneum of mice and examining the peritoneal fluid 7 to 10 days later.

Etiology and pathogenesis

Toxoplasmosis is caused by *Toxoplasma gondii*, an intracellular protozoan that requires an animal host such as a cat or sheep, in addition to the intermediate human host. Infection is caused by ingestion of cysts via food contaminated by feces of an animal host.

Treatment

No treatment is required in mild cases because toxoplasmosis is a self-limiting disease in persons with healthy immune systems.

Pyrimethamine and sulfadiazine can be given for severe cases, and the patient should be treated for up to 1 month. Spiramycin can be given as an alternative to pyrimethamine during pregnancy (due to its teratogenic effects).

Strict hygiene when handling animals is essential for prevention of the disease.

Leptospirosis

Leptospirosis is a zoonosis caused by the gram-negative organism *Leptospira interrogans*, of which there are more than 200 serotypes. It is often referred to as "Weil's disease," but this eponym should be limited to those cases of severe disease manifesting as jaundice, hemorrhage, and renal failure.

Clinical features

The clinical features of leptospirosis include acute systemic infection (i.e., fever, arthralgia, headache, anorexia).

Jaundice, hepatomegaly, renal failure, skin rash, and hemolytic anemia occur in 10–15% of cases.

Diagnosis and evaluation

The rise in liver transaminase levels may be small. Blood, cerebrospinal fluid, and urine cultures can be used to isolate the organism. A complement fixation test can be used, and specific rising titers of IgM antibody are diagnostic.

Etiology and pathogenesis

The majority of cases are due to the serotype *L. icterohaemorrhagiae*, excreted by rats in their

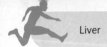

urine. Other *Leptospira* species are found in the urine of cattle, dogs, and pigs.

Infective organisms gain access via abrasions in the skin or mucous membrane, and persons particularly at risk are sewer workers, spelunkers, and persons who participate in water sports.

Complications
Renal and hepatic failure are seen in severe cases of leptospirosis. Meningitis and myocarditis occur rarely.

Prognosis
Mortality can be as high as 20%, especially in elderly persons.

Treatment
Penicillin is an effective antibiotic. Alternatively, erythromycin and tetracycline can be used. Doxycycline provides useful prophylaxis for high-risk groups.

Brucellosis
Incidence
Brucellosis is extremely rare in the United States; it is more commonly found in countries where raw, unpasteurized milk is consumed. A diagnosis of brucellosis should be considered in persons with prolonged fever of an unknown cause.

Clinical features
The symptoms of an acute brucellosis infection are often nonspecific and insidious:
- Fever.
- Arthralgia.
- Weight loss.
- Headache.
- Night sweats.

Hepatomegaly and lymphadenopathy are commonly seen.

In chronic infection, the symptoms may persist for several months with bouts of fever and splenomegaly. Chronic derangements of liver biochemistry may be seen.

Diagnosis and evaluation
Tests to consider include the following:
- Blood culture results are positive during acute infections in approximately half of patients. Rising titers are diagnostic.

- Liver biopsy may reveal presence of granulomas, but these are nonspecific for brucellosis.

Etiology and pathogenesis
Brucellosis is a zoonosis due to a coccobacillus largely spread by ingestion of unpasteurized milk. Three species are recognized: *Brucella abortus* (which infect cattle), *Brucella melitensis* (goats and sheep), and *Brucella suis* (pigs).

The organisms travel via the lymphatics and infect lymph nodes and reticuloendothelial systems. Hypersensitivity may account for the formation of granulomas.

Treatment
A prolonged course of tetracycline and rifampicin is given. Alternatively, a combination of trimethoprim and sulfamethoxazole (co-trimoxazole) can be used.

Metabolic and genetic liver disease

In general, the following conditions often progress to chronic liver disease but are considered separately here.

Nonalcoholic fatty liver disease
Nonalcoholic fatty liver disease (NAFLD) is an increasingly prevalent problem in the world. This is a spectrum of disease ranging from fatty liver (steatosis), nonalcoholic steatohepatitis (NASH), fibrosis, and finally cirrhosis. The risk factors for NAFLD include obesity, diabetes mellitus, and hyperlipidemia. The histologic changes of NASH are similar to alcoholic hepatitis, and only a careful history that excludes alcoholism will aid in a firm diagnosis. When patients develop cirrhosis, fatty changes may disappear from liver biopsy and hence may be diagnosed as cryptogenic cirrhosis. There is no effective treatment for NAFLD. Weight reduction, treatment of hyperlipidemia, and better control of diabetes mellitus are recommended.

Hemochromatosis
Incidence
Hemochromatosis is an autosomal recessive disorder caused by excess iron accumulation affecting approximately 0.5% of the white population, with a heterozygote frequency of up to 10%. Phenotypic expression of the disease is uncommon.

Clinical features

The features of hemochromatosis are dependent on patient sex, dietary intake, age, and associated toxins (e.g., alcohol) (Fig. 18.10). Men tend to present up to a decade earlier due to the protective mechanism of menstrual blood loss in women. In developing countries, iron deficiency and hookworm infestation can result in later manifestation of organ damage.

Patients may rarely present between the fourth and fifth decades of life with the classic triad of:

- Skin pigmentation (melanin deposition).
- Diabetes mellitus ("bronze diabetes").
- Hepatomegaly, if the iron deposition is severe.

Other common presentations include gonadal atrophy and loss of libido resulting from pituitary dysfunction, cardiac failure, arthritis in small joints of the hand, and chondrocalcinosis in the knees.

Diagnosis and evaluation

Relevant test results include the following:

- Serum iron is usually elevated with a low total iron-binding capacity in the presence of hemochromatosis.
- Transferrin saturation is elevated (often 100%; normal, <50%). In a fasting state, this elevation is highly suggestive of hemochromatosis.

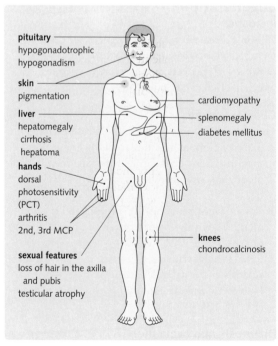

Fig. 18.10 Body map for hemochromatosis (MCP, metacarpophalangeal joint; PCT, porphyria cutanea tarda).

- The serum ferritin level is usually grossly elevated (>1000 µg/L; normal, <300 in males and <200 in females) in the presence of hemochromatosis. Ferritin levels can also be elevated in rheumatoid or other inflammatory diseases or in alcoholic liver disease, as it is an acute-phase protein.
- A hemochromatosis gene test is useful in the surveillance of family members.
- Liver biopsy is the definitive diagnostic test for hemochromatosis and also provides an assessment of the extent of liver damage. Increased parenchymal iron deposition is also seen in alcoholic cirrhosis. Iron is demonstrated by Perls' potassium cyanide stain, producing a Prussian blue appearance if hemosiderin iron is present. Iron deposition is graded I through IV, depending on degree and distribution. Grades III and IV are usually diagnostic of hemochromatosis. A hepatic iron index of more than 1.9 (mg iron per mg dry weight liver divided by the patient's age in years) is also diagnostic and is useful for differentiating genetic hemochromatosis from iron loading in alcoholic liver disease.
- The fasting blood glucose level should be measured to exclude secondary diabetes mellitus from the diagnosis.
- An electrocardiogram and echocardiogram should be undertaken to detect evidence of cardiomyopathy.

Etiology and pathogenesis

In the normal physiologic state, iron absorption is regulated in the proximal small intestine according to the body's requirements. In hemochromatosis, the regulatory mechanism is faulty, leading to inappropriate levels of absorption even when iron stores are excessive.

The condition is characterized by increased deposition in the liver parenchymal cells, in which extensive pigmentation and fibrosis develop and eventually cirrhosis occurs.

Increased iron content also occurs in endocrine glands, the heart, and skin.

Iron accumulation is gradual throughout life, and there is a threshold below which tissue damage may not occur (e.g., 5 mg/g in the liver), hence the late presentation.

C282Y and H63D mutations on chromosome 6 account for the vast majority (>85%) of cases of hemochromatosis. Patients who are homozygous for

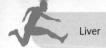

C282Y or have compound heterozygosity (one allele of each mutation, C282Y/H63D) are prone to develop hemochromatosis. However, presence of these mutations does not indicate disease because phenotypic expression is highly variable.

Complications

If untreated, cirrhosis is a common end point of hemochromatosis. This is followed by liver failure, which may be accompanied by portal hypertension.

Up to one third of male patients who have cirrhosis may develop hepatocellular carcinoma (Fig. 18.11).

Treating patients reverses the tissue damage and improves the survival rate. However, the risk of malignant change may persist if cirrhosis is already present.

It is imperative to screen first-degree relatives for the condition before the development of irreversible liver damage. This can be achieved by checking serum ferritin levels or by attempting to identify the culpable gene. Genetic testing is more useful in first-degree relatives to predict risk, even if ferritin levels are normal. Genetic testing for other subgroups has not been widely adopted because, although the condition tends to run "true" in families, the phenotypic expression of the homozygous state in the wider population is variable (i.e., only a proportion of persons homozygous for the mutation will develop iron overload). Biochemical testing with serum ferritin or transferrin saturation is usually used more for screening the population.

Aims and indications for treatment

The goals of treatment are to reduce body iron stores (reflected by serum ferritin levels) to within normal levels and limit the progression of liver damage and other affected organs in all patients who have a positive diagnosis of hemochromatosis.

Treatment plan

Treatment should consist of:

- Venesection. One unit of blood (450 mL) contains approximately 250 mg of iron. Weekly venesection is required for 6 to 12 months to remove the 20 to 40 g of excess iron present. Regular removal of 2 to 3 units of blood per year thereafter maintains ferritin levels within normal limits.
- Chelating agents (e.g., desferrioxamine) for patients who cannot tolerate venesection. Ascorbic

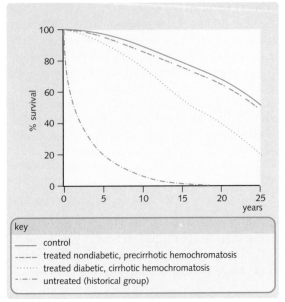

Fig. 18.11 Survival with iron overload depends on the development of complications. Even so, depletion of iron stores prolongs survival. Life expectancy is normal if treatment is started before the onset of end-organ damage.

key
— control
---- treated nondiabetic, precirrhotic hemochromatosis
······ treated diabetic, cirrhotic hemochromatosis
-·-·- untreated (historical group)

acid supplements should be avoided by these patients because it enhances iron absorption.

Wilson's disease (hepatolenticular degeneration)
Incidence

Wilson's disease is a rare inborn error of copper metabolism affecting approximately 3 in 100,000 persons with pockets of higher prevalence in Northern India and Sicily.

Clinical features

The clinical features of Wilson's disease include:

- Signs of chronic liver disease with a neurologic manifestation of basal ganglia damage (i.e., tremor, dysarthria, choreoathetosis, and eventually dementia).
- Kayser-Fleischer copper brown ring in Descemet's membrane in the cornea (often requires slit lamp to see).
- Renal tubular damage giving rise to renal tubular acidosis and renal failure, if severe.
- Hemolytic anemia and osteoporosis in rare cases (Fig. 18.12).

Diagnosis and evaluation

Wilson's disease should be suspected in young patients who present with hemolysis, jaundice, and

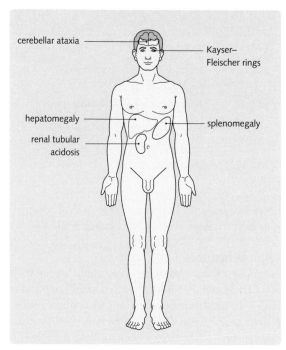

cerebellar ataxia

Kayser–
Fleischer rings

hepatomegaly

splenomegaly

renal tubular
acidosis

Fig. 18.12 Body map for Wilson's disease.

disproportionately low alkaline phosphatase levels. Serum copper and ceruloplasmin levels are usually low or normal. The urinary copper level is grossly elevated in 24-hour collection (>10 times the normal range).

A definitive diagnosis depends on a liver biopsy and the amount of copper deposition, although elevated copper levels in the liver are found in chronic cholestasis.

Etiology and pathogenesis
Wilson's disease is due to an autosomal recessive gene located on chromosome 13. There are at least 30 mutations described resulting in a faulty transporter protein (ATP7B) that excretes copper from the liver via the Golgi complex. The export of copper stimulates ceruloplasmin synthesis, hence the explanation for its low levels in Wilson's disease.

Complications
Complications may include:
- Cirrhosis, with ensuing liver failure if left untreated.
- Neurologic manifestations, which can be severe and disabling.
- Metabolic consequences of renal tubular acidosis and potentially renal failure.

Prognosis
Early diagnosis and treatment can lessen the risk of mortality and morbidity considerably, but once neurologic features are established, they are often irreversible.

Aims and indications for treatment
All patients with Wilson's disease are treated to reduce copper deposition and to avoid life-threatening complications.

Treatment plan
Lifelong oral intake of penicillamine is an effective treatment, but serious side effects can occur, limiting its usage. Blood disorders, including thrombocytopenia, agranulocytosis, and aplastic anemia can occur. Proteinuria, associated with immune complex nephritis, occurs in up to one third of patients but may resolve despite continuation of treatment. Complete blood count and urine testing for blood and protein should be undertaken frequently, particularly after the initiation of treatment. Urine copper levels should be monitored. All first-degree relatives should be screened for early treatment.

Penicillamine and trientene (triethylamine) are copper-chelating agents that have been shown to be effective. They increase urinary copper excretion but do not completely ''decopper'' the liver, instead causing the copper to be associated with metallothionein protein. Zinc treatment is also effective in reducing copper absorption and increasing metallothionein synthesis.

Alpha–1-antitrypsin deficiency
Incidence
Alpha–1-antitrypsin deficiency is inherited as a rare autosomal recessive disorder. Alpha–1-antitrypsin is a protease inhibitor produced in the liver that mediates various inflammatory processes.

Clinical features
Typical symptoms of alpha–1-antitrypsin deficiency include:
- Late-onset liver cirrhosis (in persons older than 50 years).
- Early onset of pulmonary basal emphysema (5% of homozygotes by the age of 40 years).

135

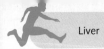

Diagnosis and evaluation

Appropriate tests include:

- Low-serum alpha–1-antitrypsin level.
- Liver biopsy to monitor for changes of cirrhosis with periodic acid-Schiff–positive staining globules within hepatocytes.
- Genotype testing. Depending on the amino acid mutation, various levels of severity of the disease can occur (i.e., those with genotype ZZ have the worse prognosis) (Fig. 18.13). Only those homozygous (PiZZ) for alpha–1-antitrypsin deficiency are proven to manifest the disease.
- Chest radiograph and pulmonary function tests to identify evidence of emphysema.

Etiology and pathogenesis

The gene responsible for alpha–1-antitrypsin deficiency is located on chromosome 14. The variant of alpha–1-antitrypsin is characterized by position on an electrophoretic strip (i.e., M, medium; S, slow; and Z, very slow).

- The normal genotype is MM. S and Z variants are due to a single polypeptide mutation, resulting in reduced synthesis and secretion of normal alpha–1-antitrypsin. S produces approximately 60% of the activity produced by M and only 15% of that produced by Z.
- Clinical phenotypes can be homozygous (e.g., ZZ) or compound heterozygous (e.g., MZ, MS, SZ).

Complications

Liver and respiratory failure due to cirrhosis and basal emphysema, respectively, usually occur.

Prognosis

Up to 15% of patients with ZZ genotype will develop cirrhosis by the fifth decade of life, and 5% will develop emphysema by the fourth decade.

Treatment plan

There are no specific treatments available for alpha–1-antitrypsin deficiency. Treatments for chronic liver disease apply. Patients with hepatic failure should be considered for liver transplantation. Smoking should be stopped because it results in up to a four-fold increase in the rate of decline of the forced expiratory volume in 1 second.

Cystic fibrosis
Incidence

More patients with cystic fibrosis are now surviving into adolescence and adulthood, and the incidence of

Alpha-1-antitrypsin deficiency	
PiMM	Normal phenotype
PiMZ	Heterozygous for alpha-1-antitrypsin deficiency (variable type)
PiSZ	Heterozygous for alpha-1-antitrypsin deficiency
PiZZ	Homozygous for alpha-1-antitrypsin deficiency (severe type)

Fig. 18.13 Variants in alpha–1-antitrypsin deficiency (Pi, protease inhibitor).

liver complications has risen. Up to 10% of patients may have established cirrhosis by their mid–20s.

Clinical features

Newborn infants with cystic fibrosis may present with obstructive jaundice in the first few weeks of life due to the accumulation of viscous secretions in a similar fashion to meconium ileus. Recovery is usual within 6 months, but some will die of hepatic failure in infancy.

In those who survive, symptomatic liver disease can be seen in up to 15% of adolescents.

Etiology and pathogenesis

Cystic fibrosis is thought to be due to obstruction of the biliary tree by mucus plugs, but the lesions can be patchy and can be missed on liver biopsy. Liver cirrhosis occurs in most cases in those with hepatic involvement.

Portal hypertension and splenomegaly may occur as a consequence of liver cirrhosis.

Prognosis

It is now recognized that the underlying liver disease is a significant prognostic factor for overall survival in cystic fibrosis. Patients with marked liver impairment have a worse outcome that may influence the timing of transplantation.

Treatment

The treatment of cirrhosis is the same regardless of the underlying etiology. Patients who are suitable may be considered for heart/lung/liver transplant, which will significantly improve their outcome (Fig. 18.14).

Chronic liver disease

This section deals predominantly with chronic liver disease with an autoimmune basis. Other causes of

Interpretation of autoantibody tests in liver disease					
Antibody	Inference	ALT, AST elevation	Alk Phos, GGT elevation	Raised immunoglobulins	Diagnostic test
AMA	PBC	Slight	Moderate	Mainly IgM, some IgG	AMA-M$_2$ subtype, liver biopsy
SMA, ANF, LKM	AICAH	Moderate	Slight	Mainly IgG	Liver biopsy
pANCA	PSC	Slight	Moderate	Some IgG	ERCP

Fig. 18.18 Comparison of antibody profiles in autoimmune liver disease (Alk Phos, alkaline phosphatase; GGT, gamma-glutamyl transferase; AMA, antimitochondrial antibody; PBC, primary biliary cirrhosis; SMA, smooth muscle antibody; ANF, antinuclear antibody; LKM, liver kidney microsomal antibody; AICAH, autoimmune chronic active hepatitis; pANCA, antineutrophil cytoplasmic antibody; PSC, primary sclerosing cholangitis; ERCP, endoscopic retrograde cholangiopancreatography).

Complications

Complications associated with autoimmune chronic active hepatitis include cirrhosis and liver failure. Patients are also more likely to develop other organ-specific autoimmune diseases.

Prognosis

A pattern of remission and exacerbation for several years followed by cirrhosis is characteristic. Half will die within 5 years if no treatment is given, compared with a 90% survival rate with treatment.

Aims and indications for treatment

Early diagnosis and prompt treatment are paramount to lessen the risk of mortality and morbidity.

Treatment plan

Corticosteroids to induce biochemical and histologic remission, with subsequent addition of azathioprine (an antiproliferative immunosuppressant) as a steroid-sparing agent, is the adopted treatment strategy.

Sarcoidosis and liver

Sarcoidosis is a chronic, multisystem disease characterized by the presence of noncaseating granulomas that predominantly affect the lung, lymph nodes, and skin, but the liver is also affected (rarely). Cardiac, renal, and neurologic manifestations are also seen.

The underlying etiology is unknown, and the majority of cases present as an incidental finding of bilateral hilar lymphadenopathy.

Autoimmune chronic active hepatitis is a rare cause of hepatosplenomegaly, producing portal hypertension either as a direct consequence of the granulomas compressing the portal venules or periportal scarring resulting in obstruction.

In cases of difficulty in diagnosing systemic sarcoidosis, a liver biopsy may be diagnostic, especially in the presence of abnormal liver enzymes. Serum angiotensin-converting enzyme levels are often elevated but not diagnostic, and those are more useful in monitoring disease activity. A Kveim skin test (still rarely performed by dermatologists) is positive.

Hepatic complications are those of portal hypertension with or without decompensated liver disease.

Systemic steroids are not beneficial in cases of hepatic sarcoidosis and are not indicated unless used for concomitant disease affecting other organ systems. Methotrexate and corticosteroids are used for the treatment of granulomatous hepatitis of unclear etiology.

Alcoholic liver disease
Incidence and diagnosis

Approximately 1% of the population is psychologically or physically dependent on alcohol:

- Twenty to thirty percent of these develop alcoholic liver disease.
- Approximately 25% of liver cirrhosis is due to alcohol.

Current recommendations for safe alcohol consumption are 21 (male) and 14 (female) units per week.

- A unit of alcohol (approximately 10 g) represents a measure of spirit, a glass of wine, or half pint of beer (see Fig. 21.3).
- An intake of 20 units (or more) per day is associated with a high risk of hepatocellular damage.

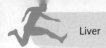

Clinical features

Diagnosis of alcoholic liver disease is made predominantly on clinical grounds, and the extent of liver damage can be determined by liver biopsy but does not always correlate well with deranged liver biochemistry.

Symptoms can often be vague, including nausea, vomiting, abdominal pain, and diarrhea, and may be attributable to the effects of alcohol or alcohol withdrawal. More extensive hepatocellular damage may manifest from jaundice to hepatic failure.

Extrahepatic manifestations include:
• Wernicke's and Korsakoff's syndromes.
• Proximal myopathy.
• Peripheral neuropathy (often painful).
• Cardiomyopathy, with cardiac failure and arrythmias.
• Gastritis and erosions.
• Porphyria cutanea tarda.
• Neglect and malnutrition.
• Psychosocial difficulties.

The CAGE questionnaire is a quick assessment for evidence of a dependency on alcohol. Ask patients whether they have ever:
• **C**ut down on alcohol for any reason.
• Become **A**ngry when people discuss their alcohol consumption.
• Felt **G**uilty because of their alcohol consumption.
• Needed an **E**ye-opener early in the day to help them cope.

Pathogenesis

Three main types of liver damage are described:
• Fatty change.
• Alcoholic hepatitis.
• Fibrosis.

Fatty change

Ethanol is metabolized in the liver, which results in hepatic fatty acid synthesis and reduced fatty acid oxidation leading to accumulation and fatty destruction of the hepatic cells (Fig. 18.19). Similar changes can also be seen in obesity, diabetes, starvation, and pregnancy.

There is thought to be no permanent hepatocellular damage, hence fatty change resolves with abstinence from alcohol.

Alcoholic hepatitis

Infiltration with polymorphonuclear leucocytes and hyaline material (Mallory bodies) is typical. Fatty change often coexists with alcoholic hepatitis. Mallory bodies may also be seen in this form of chronic active hepatitis; they are not specific to alcoholic damage.

Fibrosis

Presence of fibrosis with nodular regeneration implies previous or continuing liver damage. A micronodular pattern progresses to macronodular in later stages.

Diagnosis and evaluation

A background of chronic liver disease and a history of heavy alcohol consumption are highly indicative of alcoholic liver disease.

Other investigations may aid diagnosis:
• Complete blood count often reveals a macrocytosis, a sensitive indicator of heavy alcohol consumption. Iron-deficiency anemia may be seen in cases of chronic gastrointestinal (GI) bleed due to varices or gastric or esophageal erosion. Leukocytosis is common. Thrombocytopenia occurs as a result of the toxic effect of ethanol on megakaryocytes.
• Liver biochemistry: gamma glutamyl transferase is another indicator of heavy alcohol intake. In the presence of hepatitis, raised AST, ALT, bilirubin, and alkaline phosphatase levels will be seen. The AST level is usually only moderately raised at levels below 300 IU/L; ALT is usually less than half that value, and it has been suggested that the AST:ALT ratio is a useful indicator of alcoholic liver disease when in excess of 2. Low albumin may suggest underlying cirrhosis and impaired synthetic function. Zieve syndrome is a triad of jaundice, hyperlipidemia, and hemolytic anemia in patients with alcoholic liver disease.
• A clotting screen may reveal a prolonged prothrombin time, which is typical of alcoholic hepatitis due to reduced production of clotting factors by the liver.

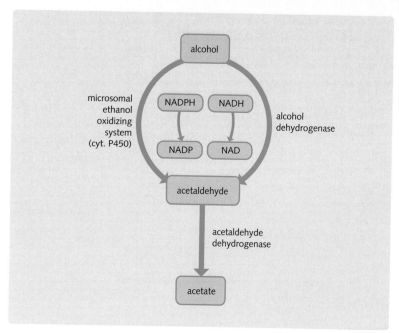

Fig. 18.19 Biochemical pathways for the metabolism of alcohol. Under normal circumstances, alcohol is converted to acetaldehyde by the action of alcohol dehydrogenase. In heavy drinkers, induction of the cytochrome P450 enzyme system occurs, hence increasing the metabolism of alcohol. Free radicals are a by-product of NADP and NAD production, causing hepatocellular damage (NAD, nicotinamide adenine dinucleotide; NADP, nicotinamide adenine dinucleotide phosphate; NADH, dihydronicotinomide adenine dinucleotide; NADPH, dihydronicotinomide adenine dinucleotide phosphate).

- Ultrasound will demonstrate fatty change and, if there is macronodular cirrhosis, may demonstrate an irregular margin with irregular intrahepatic foci mimicking metastatic disease.
- Liver biopsy is the gold standard of diagnosis. Difficulty may arise due to deranged clotting, and a transjugular liver biopsy may be necessary to reduce the bleeding risk. Features of fatty change and cirrhosis will be seen. End-stage cirrhosis seen on histology will not distinguish its underlying etiology.

Complications

Complications associated with alcoholic liver disease include liver failure and cirrhosis.

Prognosis

The prognosis is dependent on abstinence. Patients without established cirrhosis have a 5-year survival rate of 60% if they continue to drink alcohol, which rises to 90% if they discontinue. Cirrhotic patients who continue to drink alcohol have an even poorer prognosis, with a 5-year survival rate of 35%.

Treatment of alcoholic hepatitis

Abstinence from alcohol is vital. Acute alcohol withdrawal (i.e., hallucinations, tremor, fits, and delirium tremens) should be treated with a decrementing regimen of a benzodiazepine such as diazepam or chlordiazepoxide. Multivitamins, especially vitamin B complex, should be given in addition to high-protein and high-calorie supplements, except in cases of hepatic encephalopathy.

The treatment of alcoholic hepatitis is mostly symptomatic and includes nutritional support and alcohol abstinence. Patients with hepatic encephalopathy and those with a discriminant function (DF) score greater than 32 may benefit from prednisone, and the patient may be given a trial of prednisone if there is no evidence of infection. A DF score greater than 32 is associated with a mortality rate of approximately 50%. [The DF score formula is $4.6 \times$ (patient's PT − control PT) + total bilirubin (mg/dL).] Pentoxifylline has also been found to be beneficial in one study, but this needs further confirmation.

Cirrhosis

Cirrhosis is the end stage of any progressive liver disease.

Clinical features

Cirrhosis per se is usually asymptomatic. Symptoms arise due to either the underlying disease or when complications of cirrhosis ensue.

143

Abdominal examination may reveal:
- Hepatomegaly or splenomegaly (if portal hypertension is present).
- Ascites.
- Dilated umbilical veins (caput medusae; Fig. 18.20).

Stigmata of chronic liver disease in the skin include anemia, jaundice, palmar erythema, Dupuytren's contracture, finger clubbing, leukonychia, pruritus, spider nevi, and xanthomas.

There may be endocrine features such as loss of hair, testicular atrophy, parotid enlargement, gynecomastia, amenorrhea, and loss of libido (see Fig. 18.20).

Neurologic features include drowsiness, confusion, flapping of hands, constructional apraxia, and fetor hepaticus (portosystemic encephalopathy).

Fluid retention may be apparent in the abdomen (ascites) or as peripheral edema.

Evaluation

Tests to consider include the following:
- Liver biochemistry results can be surprisingly normal, but some abnormality will often be present with slightly raised transaminase and alkaline phosphatase levels. In severe cases, all liver enzyme counts will be abnormal. Low sodium and albumin levels are also seen. Hyperglycemia can be evident if there is associated pancreatic insufficiency, and hypertriglyceridemia is common.
- A complete blood count may reveal anemia due to variceal bleeding. Macrocytosis can be a direct effect of alcohol, in addition to vitamin B_{12} or folate deficiency.
- Coagulopathy is a very sensitive indicator of liver dysfunction and is reflected in the prolonged prothrombin time.
- Alpha-fetoprotein is raised in hepatocellular carcinoma (although it can be slightly elevated with cirrhosis—serial measurements are useful).
- Ultrasound provides information of liver size, fatty change, and fibrosis as well as hepatocellular carcinoma.
- Endoscopy identifies and allows treatment for varices.
- Liver biopsy may be indicated for patients in whom the underlying etiology is unclear or to assess the severity of cirrhosis.

Other tests (e.g., hepatitis serology, ferritin, ceruloplasmin, autoantibodies) are useful in establishing the underlying etiology.

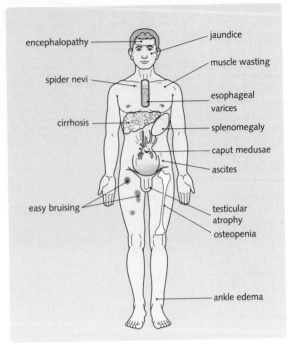

Fig. 18.20 Body map showing features of cirrhosis.

Etiology and pathogenesis

Cirrhosis of the liver is a result of cell necrosis followed by fibrosis and regeneration, hence the formation of nodules (Fig. 18.21).

The most common causes worldwide are chronic hepatitis B and C infections and alcohol.
- Cirrhosis is the result of fibrosis and regeneration with distortion of hepatic architecture and resultant nodule formation. The nodules have been characterized by size as micronodular and macronodular cirrhosis based on gross appearance, although the appearance is not reliably indicative of underlying etiology. The size of the nodule depends on the duration of cirrhosis.

Complications
Portal hypertension

Portal hypertension results from an increase in the vascular resistance due to anatomic changes (e.g., collagen deposition, fibrosis and cirrhosis, contraction of myofibroblasts) and an upregulation of vasoconstrictors. This leads to the formation of gastroesophageal varices (see Fig. 18.20). In addition, sodium retention and vasoactive substances such as

A	Causes of cirrhosis
Alcohol excess	
Chronic viral hepatitis, especially B and C	
Genetic diseases (e.g., hemochromatosis, alpha–1-antitrypsin deficiency, Wilson's disease)	
Chronic liver diseases (e.g., primary biliary cirrhosis, autoimmune chronic hepatitis)	
Cryptogenic where no etiology is apparent. NAFLD is the most likely cause.	

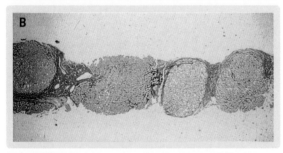

Fig. 18.21 A. Common causes of cirrhosis (NAFLD, nonalcoholic fatty liver disease). B. Low-power photomicrograph of needle liver biopsy showing fibrous nodular formation and established cirrhosis.

nitric oxide (due to an accumulation of toxic metabolites) will increase plasma volume and splanchnic vasodilatation, respectively, and thus maintain portal hypertension.

Bleeding from the varices will result in hematemesis and melena and can be precipitated by trauma (e.g., food bolus) or rising portal venous pressure (i.e., progressive liver cirrhosis).

Ascites

Ascites is a result of fluid in the peritoneal cavity, and its pathogenesis involves several physiologic processes.

Sodium and water retention occur as a result of activation of the renin-angiotensin system, secondary to arterial vasodilatation (caused by vasoactive substances such as nitric oxide). Portal hypertension per se results in a high serum and ascites albumin gradient due to increased hydrostatic pressure; hence, it further reduces intravascular volume and stimulates sodium and water retention via aldosterone (secondary hyperaldosteronism).

Ascites may be aggravated by a low plasma oncotic pressure resulting from hypoalbuminenia, which occurs as a result of impaired synthetic hepatic function.

Spontaneous bacterial infection of ascites is a serious complication that carries a significant risk of mortality (50%). Common pathogens include *Escherichia coli*, *Klebsiella* species, and other gut bacteria. Clinical deterioration (often nonspecific), fever, and neutrophilia should raise the possibility of infected ascites. Aspiration of ascitic fluid should be performed for Gram stain and culture. Treatment with broad-spectrum antibiotics such as a third-generation cephalosporin (e.g., cefotaxime) should be employed.

Hepatic encephalopathy

Toxic metabolites that are usually detoxified by the liver accumulate in the bloodstream and pass through the blood-brain barrier to cause encephalopathy. Ammonia produced by the breakdown of proteins initiated by intestinal bacteria appears to play a role in hepatic encephalopathy. The accumulation of false neurotransmitters is also important, though poorly understood.

Clinically, the patient is confused and disoriented and has slurred speech and, in severe cases, convulsion and coma. Coarse flapping of hyperextended hands (i.e., asterixis), hepatic fetor (i.e., sweet-smelling breath due to ketones), and constructional apraxia (i.e., patient is unable to draw a five-pointed star) can also be seen.

Acute onset usually has a precipitating factor that can potentially be reversible (e.g., bleeding or infection).

Hepatorenal syndrome

Hepatorenal syndrome (HRS) is diagnosed in patients with cirrhosis when serum creatinine is at least 1.5 mg/dL in the absence of hypovolemia, sepsis, other precipitating factors (e.g., drugs), or intrinsic renal disease. A fluid challenge is recommended before HRS is diagnosed. There are two types of HRS:
- Type II HRS involves a slow increase of serum creatinine to 1.5 mg/dL or more.
- Type I HRS involves the doubling of serum creatinine over a period of 2 weeks.

Type I HRS is associated with a very poor prognosis, and most patients die within a month if they did not receive liver transplantation. There is no effective treatment for HRS apart from liver transplantation.

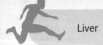

It is thought to be due to a depletion in intravascular volume, activation of the renin-angiotensin system, and vasoconstriction of the renal afferent arterioles—hence, reduced glomerular filtration.

Other mediators have also been implicated that are related to prostaglandin synthesis, and the syndrome can be precipitated by the use of nonsteroidal anti-inflammatory drugs. More commonly, renal impairment occurs as a result of sepsis, diuretic use, or excessive paracentesis causing intravascular volume depletion and renal hypoperfusion.

The renal abnormality is thought to be functional because transplanted kidneys from a donor patient with HRS to a recipient will result in a normal functioning kidney. However, extreme cases will cause tubular necrosis and renal damage.

Hepatocellular carcinoma

The development of cirrhosis is an independent risk factor for hepatocellular carcinoma (see section Tumors of the liver starting on p. 150).

Prognosis

The 5-year survival rate for persons with hepatocellular carcinoma is dependent on the severity of liver disease; Childs class C cirrhosis (Fig. 18.22) or those with very high Model of End-Stage Liver Disease (MELD) scores have very poor prognosis. MELD score is calculated using a mathematical formula (MELD score = $3.8 * \log_e(\text{bilirubin [mg/dL]}) + 11.2 * \log_e(\text{INR}) + 9.6 * \log_e(\text{creatinine [mg/dL]}) + 6.4$) that uses serum bilirubin, serum creatinine, and the international normalized ratio (INR; http://www.unos.org); recently, MELD score has been shown to be an accurate predictor of short-term mortality and is currently used for organ allocation in the United States.

Treatment

Treatment generally consists of managing the complications that arise.

If ascites is present, spontaneous bacterial infection must be excluded; if infection is found, appropriate therapy should be started.

A reduction in dietary sodium (sodium less than 2000 mg/day) will allow the reabsorption of ascitic fluid back into the circulation.

Modified Childs classification			
Childs class points	0	1	2
Bilirubin	<2 mg/dL	2–3 mg/dL	>3 mg/dL
Albumin	>3.5 g/dL	2.8–3.6 g/dL	<2.8 mg/dL
INR	<1.7	1.8–2.3 or PT 4 sec above normal	>2.3 or PT 5 sec above normal
Ascites	None	Minimal or controlled with therpay	Moderate or marked or refractory to therapy
Encephalopathy	None	Minimal	>Grade II

Childs class A = 5 or 6 points; class B = 7 to 9 points; class C = 10 or more points.

Modifications in serum bilirubin are made for cholestatic liver diseases.

Fig. 18.22 Modified Childs classification of cirrhosis based on functional capacity of the liver. Class C carries a poor prognosis (INR, international normlized ratio; PT, prothrombin time).

Diuretic therapy is used to increase renal excretion of sodium and hence excess water. Hepatic dysfunction results in secondary hyperaldosteronism because of a failure to break down aldosterone in the liver. Spironolactone, a specific aldosterone antagonist, is therefore the diuretic of choice. Further diuresis may be required, and the use of a loop diuretic such as furosemide (frusemide) is effective, but the patient is at risk of hyponatremia, dehydration, and hypokalemia. Paracentesis is often carried out for symptomatic relief.

Various shunts can be inserted for persistent ascites such that they drain peritoneal fluid into the internal jugular vein, but infection and blockage of the shunts limit their use.

Paracentesis should be limited to 8 to 10 L per session with concomitant administration of albumin at 6 to 8 g/L of fluid removed. Albumin or other plasma expanders are used to prevent intravascular volume depletions.

A transjugular intrahepatic portosystemic shunt (TIPS) is used effectively in patients with ascites that is refractory to medical treatment. In controlled trials, TIPS has been shown to be as effective as repeated paracentesis plus albumin infusion. The major risk of TIPS is hepatic encephalopathy.

Treatment of encephalopathy typically includes lactulose with an aim to have 2 to 3 bowel movements per day. Nonabsorbable antibiotics such as neomycin or metronidazole could be used when patients are noncompliant with lactulose or when lactulose fails to control hepatic encephalopathy adequately. A low-protein diet should be recommended only when encephalopathy becomes refractory to medical treatment.

Liver transplantation is the only definitive treatment for advanced cirrhosis. The option of transplantation should be offered to all patients with decompensated liver disease (i.e., Childs class B or C cirrhosis). Expedited transplantation is often necessary for patients with concomitant HCC, those with type I HRS or those with very high MELD scores (i.e., >30). The organ allocation system for the United States is managed by the United Network for Organ Sharing. The country is divided into 11 regions, and each region is further subdivided into organ procurement areas. The organs are allocated according to blood type and MELD scores. MELD score is used to prioritize patients on the transplant list; the score ranges from 7 to 40, with the highest priority allocated to the highest score. If there is a tie, the waiting period is considered for allocation. Survival after transplantation is excellent, with 85–90% survival at 1 year and 70–75% survival at 5 years. Many patients resume normal life and activities including full-time employment and participation in sports. Immunosuppression to prevent rejection must be maintained lifelong, but it also places the patient at increased risk of infections and malignancies. Recurrence of chronic liver diseases including viral hepatitis, primary biliary cirrhosis, or primary sclerosing cholangitis can occur and sometimes cause liver damage and cirrhosis, requiring retransplantation—especially in patients with recurrent HCV infection.

Esophageal and gastric varices
Incidence
Esophageal and gastric varices are a major complication of cirrhosis, whatever the underlying etiology. Up to 70% of patients with cirrhosis will develop varices, and up to 30% of these varices will bleed.

Portal vein thrombosis causes noncirrhotic portal hypertension.

Clinical features
Acute GI tract bleed in the form of melena or hematemesis due to rupture of varices is the usual mode of presentation. Other features may include:
- Stigmata of chronic liver disease: palmar erythema, spider nevi, proximal myopathy or muscle wasting, pigmentation or jaundice, hypogonadism.
- Splenomegaly, due to underlying portal hypertension.
- Features of liver failure (e.g., encephalopathy, ascites, jaundice).

Diagnosis and evaluation
- Appropriate tests are as follows:
- Complete blood count, biochemistry, clotting, etc., as for all patients with an acute GI tract bleed. A low platelet count may indicate hypersplenism due to portal hypertension. Prolonged prothrombin time is an indicator of diminished hepatic synthetic function.
- Urgent endoscopy is essential to confirm the diagnosis and differentiate variceal hemorrhage from other causes.
- Liver biopsy may be required after recovery from the acute episode, if the etiology of liver disease remains in doubt.
- Ultrasound and Doppler studies may be useful to diagnose hepatic or portal vein thrombosis.

Etiology and pathogenesis
Esophageal and gastric varices may be due to presence of portal hypertension, which can be:
- Presinusoidal.
- Sinusoidal.
- Postsinusoidal.

When portal pressure rises above 10 to 12 mmHg (normal, 5 to 8 mmHg), collateral communication with the systemic venous system occurs instead of blood flowing into the hepatic vein. Portosystemic anastomoses occur at the gastroesophageal junction, ileocecal junction, rectum, and anterior abdominal wall via the umbilical vein (Figs. 18.23 and 18.24).

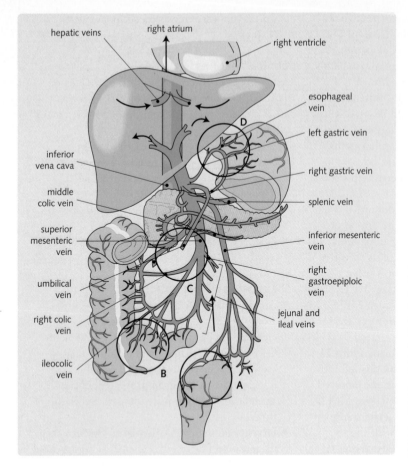

Fig. 18.23 Portal vasculature and sites of portal systemic anastomoses. Sites of portosystemic anastomoses are indicated by black circles. A. Rectal varices or hemorrhoids. B. Ileocecal varices. C. Umbilical varices (caput medusae). D. Gastroesophageal varices. Varices at the gastroesophageal junction bleed most commonly only because they traverse the greatest pressure gradient between the negative pressure in the thorax and the positive-pressure abdominal cavity.

Presinusoidal portal hypertension

Presinusoidal portal hypertension (PHTN) is a blockage of the portal vein before its entry to the liver (e.g., portal vein thrombosis as a result of congenital venous abnormality, prothrombotic states, or umbilical sepsis). Pancreatic disease is the most common cause in adults. A rare cause is schistosomiasis. Doppler studies usually identify the blockage.

Sinusoidal portal hypertension

The majority of cases of sinusoidal PHTN is due to cirrhosis, where portal vascular resistance is increased due to distorted architecture and perivenular fibrosis. This can also occur in congenital hepatic fibrosis and noncirrhotic portal hypertension, where the histology shows mild portal tract fibrosis without cirrhosis.

Postsinusoidal portal hypertension

Postsinusoidal PHTN occurs in Budd-Chiari syndrome where there is occlusion of the hepatic veins as they exit the liver. The patient usually has

a hypercoagulable state, underlying myeloproliferative disorder, or extrinsic occlusion by tumor or mass.

Portal hypertension develops if the condition becomes chronic. Other causes include constrictive pericarditis and right-sided cardiac failure.

Complications

The risk of developing encephalopathy is high with an acute variceal bleed.

Prognosis

The overall risk of recurrence after an acute episode is 80% over 2 years. Each variceal bleed carries a mortality risk of 15–40%.

Aims of treatment

The aims of treatment are resuscitation, restoration of hemodynamic stability, and arrest of variceal bleeding. Once these are successfully carried out, preventive measures should be started.

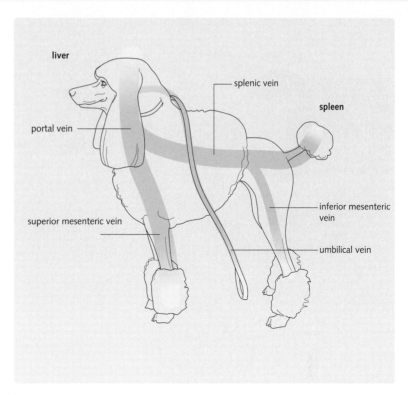

Fig. 18.24 Difficulty remembering the portal circulation? For portal, think poodle!

Treatment

Resuscitation aims to replace depleted intravascular volume with plasma expanders and crystalloids initially, then blood once available (as with all major GI tract bleeds). Correction of coagulopathy with vitamin K (takes 6 to 12 hours to work), fresh frozen plasma, or cryoprecipitate should be undertaken if required.

Urgent endoscopy is required, during which sclerosant is injected in or around the varices to cause inflammatory obliteration (see Fig. 24.18, A). Alternatively, elastic band ligation of the varices at endoscopy produces thrombotic obliteration (Fig. 18.25). Repeat banding is usually needed to prevent further bleeds. Endoscopic band ligation is preferred to sclerotherapy for prevention of variceal bleeding because of lower complication rates involving such problems as esophageal ulceration and strictures.

Vasoconstrictor agents such as octreotide (somatostatin analog) can be administered intravenously as an adjuvant therapy. The aim is to cause splanchnic vasoconstriction and hence restrict portal blood flow.

Balloon tamponade is now mainly reserved for patients for whom sclerotherapy is temporarily unavailable or in whom the procedure has failed. An inflatable tube is passed into the stomach and the balloon is inflated with air. Traction on the balloon is maintained for 12 hours until the varices have collapsed. An alternative design of the tube also has an esophageal balloon. Prolonged inflation of the balloon is associated with mucosal ulceration and rupture of the esophagus. It also increases the risk of aspiration pneumonia.

TIPS is a shunt formed between the systemic and portal venous system to treat varices (Fig. 18.26). A guidewire is passed, under X-ray control, via the internal jugular vein to the hepatic vein and into the liver. Contact is made through the liver substance with the portal venous circulation, and a metal endoprosthesis is inserted to create the shunt. Encephalopathy occurs in up to 30% of patients. Recurrence of varices can occur if the stent thromboses.

Surgery is presently rarely performed. Esophageal transection can be done as an emergency with ligation of the vessels. Portosystemic shunts (mesocaval or splenorenal) can also be undertaken surgically, but these have a high incidence of encephalopathy. Narrow-gauge stents forming a conduit between the

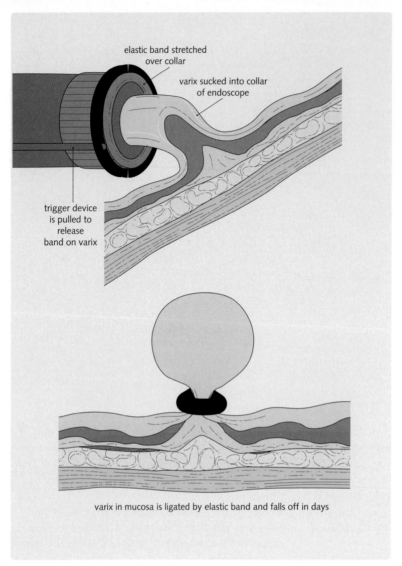

elastic band stretched over collar

varix sucked into collar of endoscope

trigger device is pulled to release band on varix

varix in mucosa is ligated by elastic band and falls off in days

Fig. 18.25 Strategy to control variceal hemorrhage by elastic band ligation.

portal vein and vena cava can improve the results but have no advantage over TIPS.

A nonselective beta-blocker (e.g., propranolol) can be given to reduce portal pressure by reducing cardiac output and allowing vasoconstriction of splanchnic arteries by inhibiting the effects of $beta_2$ receptor–mediated vasodilatation. This is the drug of choice in both primary prevention of variceal bleeding and in prevention of secondary hemorrhage after obliteration of varices. A long-acting nitrate such as isosorbide mononitrate can act as an adjuvant agent to beta blockade in reducing portal pressure.

Tumors of the liver

The most common tumors are metastatic spread from another primary site (e.g., GI tract, breast, thyroid, and bronchus). Primary tumors of the liver are usually malignant.

Hepatocellular carcinoma
Incidence
Hepatocellular carcinoma (HCC) is one of the most common malignant diseases worldwide but is rare in the Western world.

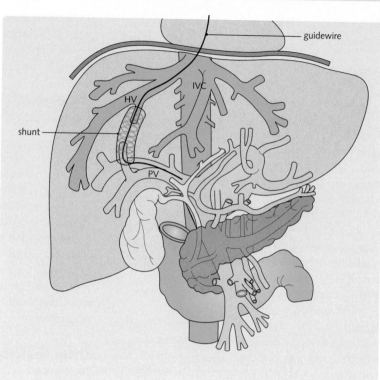

Fig. 18.26 Schematic representation of transjugular intrahepatic portocaval shunt procedure (IVC, inferior vena cava; HV, hepatic vein; PV, portal vein).

Clinical features

The clinical features of HCC are as follows:

- Symptoms are usually nonspecific (e.g., weight loss, malaise, fever, right upper quadrant pain) and, in late stages, ascites may occur.
- Cirrhotic patients who develop the above clinical features should have malignant change excluded.
- An enlarged irregular tender liver is more likely to be found in secondary metastasis or preexisting cirrhosis than primary HCC.
- Metastases to lung and bone may produce pleural effusions and pathologic fractures, respectively.

Diagnosis and evaluation

Tests to consider are as follows:

- In liver biochemistry, normal or a mild abnormality of enzyme levels is usual in established, inactive cirrhosis. A rise in ALT or AST level may be indicative of tumor necrosis. Elevated alkaline phosphatase may reflect bony metastases.
- Serum alpha-fetoprotein (AFP) is elevated only in about two thirds of patients with HCC.

An AFP level above 400 IU or a rising AFP is diagnostic of HCC. In the absence of an elevated AFP level ($\geq$400 IU), ultrasound-guided biopsy of the tumor is indicated to confirm the diagnosis.

- Ultrasound, computed tomography (CT), and magnetic resonance imaging (MRI) are used to diagnose HCC. Despite the increased sensitivity, a significant number of tumors are missed on CT or MRI. Sensitivity is lower with ultrasound, especially in inexperienced hands.
- Liver biopsy under ultrasound guidance is required for histologic diagnosis.

Etiology and pathogenesis

In areas where hepatitis B and C are prevalent, over 90% of patients with HCC have positive serology, and an equal number have preexisting cirrhosis. The etiology is presumed to be the integration of the virus into the host genome.

Most patients with cirrhosis, whatever the underlying cause, are at risk of developing HCC, especially patients with hepatitis B or C and primary hemochromatosis. Development of a hepatoma occurs more commonly in men than women with cirrhosis.

Prognosis

The prognosis of HCC is very poor; the survival rate is 5% at 6 months without treatment.

Treatment

Liver transplantation is a curative treatment for HCC, with 5-year survival reaching 70% in selected cases (small tumors without extrahepatic spread or vascular invasion). Tumors are resectable in only less than 20% of patients at presentation. Five-year survival after resection is around 40%, but 60% of patients develops recurrent HCC. Other treatment modalities include radiofrequency ablation, percutaneous ethanol injection, and transarterial chemoembolization. Often these treatments are used as a bridge while a patient is awaiting liver transplantation or as a palliative treatment. However, encouraging long-term survival rates have been reported with percutaneous ethanol injection and radiofrequency ablation in patients with small tumors and better tumor biology.

Other tumors of the liver

Adenomas

Adenomas of the liver are rare and are associated with the oral contraceptive pill. They can present as an incidental finding or due to intrahepatic bleeding. Surgical resection of hepatic adenomas is recommended since these tumors have the potential for malignant transformation.

Hemangiomas

Hemangiomas are the most common benign tumor of the liver and are usually found incidentally on ultrasound. No treatment is required. Angiography is rarely required for diagnosis because CT, MRI, or radiolabeled [99]technetium can diagnose these lesions in most cases.

Focal nodular hyperplasia

As its name suggests, focal nodular hyperplasia causes nodules in the liver, but hepatic function is normal. It is more common than hepatic adenoma but has no malignant potential. Its importance is that it can be mistaken for cirrhosis either on radiologic imaging or even on histology from a needle biopsy. It is usually asymptomatic and found incidentally but is believed to be related to the oral contraceptive pill. In these circumstances, it is thought that about 50% of patients become symptomatic, usually with pain in the right upper quadrant. Symptomatic cases are treated by surgical resection.

Drugs and the liver

Many drugs are metabolized by liver enzymes, and some are excreted in bile. Some drugs are fat-soluble, and their bioavailability can be affected by bile salt micellar concentration in the intestine. Plasma proteins, especially albumin synthesized in the liver, affect the kinetics of many drugs. Therefore, liver dysfunction and disease can impair absorption, transport, metabolism, and excretion of several drugs (Fig. 18.27). Care must be taken when using most drugs in the presence of liver disease. Conversely, many drugs can cause deranged liver biochemistry or damage.

Drug toxicity to the liver
Incidence

Up to 10% of jaundice is drug-induced and is mediated by different mechanisms.

Etiology and pathogenesis

Drug toxicity can be:

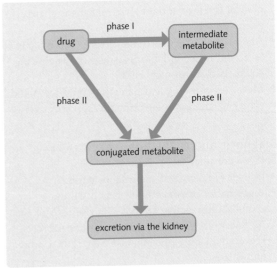

Fig. 18.27 Biochemical pathways of drug metabolism in the liver.

- Dose or duration related (e.g., azathioprine, methotrexate).
- Idiosyncratic (e.g., clavulanic acid).
- Due to overdose toxicity (e.g., acetaminophen).

Three types of pathology are described (Fig. 18.28):
- Acute hepatitis typically occurs 2 to 3 weeks after starting the drug and normally resolves after cessation. In the case of halothane, repeated exposure sensitizes the patient and can cause fulminant hepatitis, suggesting an immunologic cause. Clinically, this can mimic severe viral hepatitis.
- Cholestasis can occur; bile stasis causes a functional obstruction, hence biochemically it produces jaundice with pale stools and dark urine, usually after 4 to 6 weeks. The cause of bile stasis is unclear, but inflammatory infiltration of bile ducts and interference with excretory transport proteins have been implicated. Anabolic steroids and oral contraceptives can cause profound cholestasis.
- Necrosis can occur on a dose-dependent basis. Toxic metabolites are normally detoxified by the liver (e.g., conjugation by glutathione), and once the level of glutathione falls, toxic metabolites accumulate and liver necrosis follows. Concurrent ingestion of enzyme-inducing drugs (e.g., phenytoin, carbamazepine, and alcohol binge), severe illness, or starvation will render these persons more susceptible to toxicity.

Clinical features
The clinical features of drug toxicity can range from mild elevation of liver enzyme levels to acute fulminant hepatic failure:
- Jaundice is usually secondary to an acute hepatitis or cholestasis, but rarely it can be due to hemolysis.
- In the majority of cases, derangement of liver enzymes is found on routine examination before clinical jaundice develops.
- Nausea and vomiting or abdominal pain may occur.
- Present are pruritus, steatorrhea, and dark urine if cholestasis occurs.

Diagnosis and evaluation
Inquire carefully about the timing, chronology, and duration of drug ingestion.

Liver enzyme levels can show an acute hepatic picture (e.g., raised ALT or AST) or a cholestatic/obstructive picture (e.g., raised alkaline phosphatase and gamma glutamyl transpeptidase). Jaundice may be present in either type. It is important to establish whether there is clinical or laboratory evidence of hepatocellular dysfunction (e.g., encephalopathy, ascites, hypoalbuminemia, coagulopathy, acidosis) or associated renal impairment.

Complications and prognosis
Fulminant hepatitis secondary to halothane-induced hepatitis has a mortality rate of up to 20%, but this is rare. Hepatic failure after acute liver necrosis most often and predictably follows acetaminophen overdose.

Treatment
Withdrawal of the offending drug is usually sufficient to allow normalization of liver enzymes, within days to weeks. However, in some cases, such as chlorpromazine-induced cholestatic hepatitis, it may take up to 12 months or longer before the liver biochemistry returns to normal.

Acetaminophen toxicity
The analgesic acetaminophen is commonly used for self-poisoning, but this is a potentially treatable condition. Occasionally, overdose of acetaminophen can be accidental, or there can be a preexisting liver condition of which the patient was unaware. Unfortunately, delayed presentation can often be

Drugs affecting liver function	
Pattern of liver damage	Drugs
Hepatitis	Antituberculous: rifampin, isoniazid Antifungal: ketoconazole Antihypertensive: atenolol, verapamil Anesthetics: halothane
Cholestasis	Antiarrhythmics: amiodarone Antimetabolite: methotrexate Allopurinol Antipsychotics: chlorpromazine Antibiotics: erythromycin, clavulanic acid, flucloxacillin Immunosuppressives: cyclosporin A Contraceptives and anabolic steroids
Necrosis	Acetaminophen, carbon tetrachloride

Fig. 18.28 Drugs known to cause disturbance in liver function.

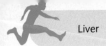
fatal. Because this is such a common and important clinical scenario, it is worth describing in detail.

Clinical features

The typical symptoms of acetaminophen toxicity are as follows:

- Nausea and vomiting usually occur within the first 24 hours.
- Liver failure can be seen within 72 to 96 hours if left untreated. Acute renal failure can occur with or without liver failure (acetaminophen can directly cause renal tubular necrosis).

Diagnosis and evaluation

Acetaminophen levels are plotted on a chart (e.g., Prescott nomogram) and correlated to "time post-ingestion" to establish the need for treatment. However, the exact timing may be difficult because the history obtained from the patient is often unreliable. If there is doubt, it is safer to initiate treatment than to wait for or rely on levels. Useful tests include:

- Clotting screen. The prothrombin time is the most sensitive indication of hepatic damage.
- Liver biochemistry. This usually shows raised ALT and AST, sometimes to very high levels (10,000), but these do not correlate well with toxicity or give any prognostic information.
- Electrolyte levels, which are usually normal. A raised creatinine level indicates significant renal damage, and a level higher than 300 μmol/L predicts a serious outcome.
- Arterial gases. A low pH (<7.3) has a significantly poorer prognosis in patients presenting late (i.e., >24 hours).
- The blood glucose level can be low, and serial measurements should be undertaken if there is evidence of hepatic failure.
- King's College criteria have been shown to accurately predict mortality in acute liver failure. In acetaminophen-induced liver failure, arterial pH lower than 7.3 or presence of grade III or IV encephalopathy plus prothrombin time greater than 100 seconds plus serum creatinine greater than 3.4 mg/dL will predict a 35% mortality rate. Similarly, in non–acetaminophen-induced liver failure, prothrombin time greater than 100 seconds or the presence of any other three prognostic predictors will predict a 95% mortality rate. Such patients should be offered liver

transplantation in an expedited fashion (Fig. 18.29).

The three most prognostically influential parameters in the setting of acetamnophen-induced acute hepatic failure are serum pH, creatinine, and prothrombin time.

Etiology and pathogenesis

Acetaminophen is converted to a toxic metabolite, N-acetyl-p-benzoquinonimine, which under normal circumstances is inactivated by conjugation with glutathione. In overdose, glutathione is depleted, hence there is a buildup of toxic metabolite, thus hepatocellular necrosis (Fig. 18.30).

Prognostic factors for acute liver failure	
Blood test/clinical signs Acetaminophen-induced failure	Mortality rate without transplantation
Arterial pH <7.3	95% without any other adverse factors
PT >100 sec (INR >6.5)	95% if all three adverse factors are present
Creatinine >3.4 mg/dL	
Stage III or IV encephalopathy	
Non–acetaminophen-induced failure	
PT >100 sec (INR >3.5)	95% without any other adverse factors
Creatinine >3.4 mg/dL	80% if one of these adverse factors is present
Bilirubin >18 mg/dL	95% if three or more of these adverse factors are present
Age <10 yr or >40 yr	
More than 7 days of jaundice before encephalopathy	
Unknown viral infections, drugs, toxins	

Fig. 18.29 Prognostic factors for acute liver failure (PT, prothrombin time; INR, international normalized ratio).

Patients with underlying liver impairment (e.g., persons with chronic alcoholism or cirrhosis) or those concurrently taking an enzyme-inducing drug (e.g., phenytoin) are at greater risk of hepatocellular damage; hence, the threshold for treatment should be lowered. Those patients with HIV are also at higher risk because they tend to have diminished stores of hepatic glutathione. There is a "high-risk" treatment line on the Prescott nomogram.

Complications

Fulminant hepatic failure is a serious and often fatal complication that is more often seen in those presenting later than 16 hours after ingestion.

Treatment

N-acetylcysteine infusion is the treatment of choice; it replenishes hepatic glutathione by providing the sulfydryl group it requires. The decision of whether treatment is required is based on serum acetaminophen levels taken 4 hours or more after ingestion, and the likelihood of severe hepatic damage is predicted. Oral methionine can be given as an alternative, but its absorption is unreliable, especially if the patient is vomiting.

Serum acetaminophen levels are unreliable in patients who present later than 16 hours after ingestion; hence, if there is any doubt, treatment should be started and stopped when subsequent liver biochemistry and clotting are found to be normal.

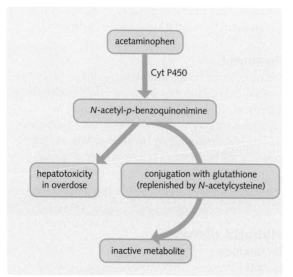

Fig. 18.30 Biochemical mechanism of acetaminophen toxicity and prevention.

Patients presenting within 1 hour of ingestion should be given activated charcoal because this will reduce the absorption of the drug from the GI tract.

Patients at risk of severe liver damage or with fulminant hepatic failure should be referred to a specialist unit for expert care and possible liver transplantation.

Prognosis

Patients who recover from hepatocellular damage do not have any residual liver impairment and can be treated as normal.

Liver abscesses

Pyogenic abscess
Incidence
Pyogenic abscess is an uncommon complication of intra-abdominal sepsis (e.g., diverticulitis, appendicitis, perforated bowel), but it can occur sporadically without any overt sign of other sources of infection.

Clinical features
The clinical features of pyogenic abscess include:
- Nonspecific symptoms such as swinging fever, anorexia, weight loss, abdominal pain, malaise.
- Jaundice, tender hepatomegaly, and septicemic shock in some cases.
- Possibly a reactive pleural effusion in the right lower lobe.

Diagnosis and evaluation
Consider the following tests to aid in diagnosis:
- Complete blood count. Normocytic normochromic anemia with neutrophilia is indicative.
- Liver biochemistry. Watch for raised alkaline phosphatase and raised bilirubin levels (if bile ducts are obstructed).
- Blood cultures. Results are positive only in approximately one third of cases. Recent antibiotic therapy reduces this further.
- Chest radiograph. A raised right hemidiaphragm with or without pleural effusion may be seen.
- Liver ultrasound. Cystic lesions (single or multiple) are seen, and ultrasound-guided aspiration of pus for microscopy and culture to identify the organism and its sensitivity.

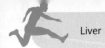

- Further imaging (e.g., CT scan of abdomen) may be required to identify the primary source of infection.

Etiology and pathogenesis

E. coli is the most common pathogen isolated. Others include *Streptococcus faecalis* (enterococcus), *Streptococcus milleri*, *Proteus* species, *Staphylococcus aureus*, and anaerobes.

Abdominal infection spread to the liver via the portovenous system is likely to be the most common cause, but direct spread from biliary infection or perinephric abscess can also occur.

Complications and prognosis

Few or no complications will occur if the pyogenic abscess is single and adequately treated. Rupture of the abscess can occur, producing bacterial peritonitis and, consequently, a significant increase in mortality.

Patients with multiple abscesses have a poorer outcome than those with a unilocular abscess, with a mortality rate of over 50% in some cases, depending on the underlying cause.

Treatment

Treatment options include the following:

- Aspiration of the abscess under ultrasound control should be done as a therapeutic intervention as well as a diagnostic procedure.
- Surgical intervention may also be required if aspiration is unsuccessful or if multiple abscesses are unsuitable for aspiration.
- Broad-spectrum antibiotics are given immediately to cover gram-positive, gram-negative, and anaerobic organisms, until sensitivity is known. A combination of benzylpenicillin, gentamicin, and metronidazole is a reasonable initial regimen.

Amebic abscess
Incidence

Amebic abscess occurs worldwide and is endemic in the tropics and subtropics.

Clinical features

The main symptoms are:

- Diarrhea as part of amebic dysentry (but not always).
- Nonspecific (e.g., malaise, anorexia, fever, abdominal pain).
- Tender hepatomegaly with or without right pleural effusion.

Rarely, clinical jaundice is seen.

Diagnosis and evaluation

Appropriate tests include:

- Liver biochemistry, which may be normal or demonstrate an isolated, raised alkaline phosphatase level.
- Blood cultures, the results of which are usually negative.
- Microscopy of stool, which may demonstrate pus, red cells, and trophozoites.
- Ameba serology (IgG). This does not indicate current disease as the results remain positive after the disease has resolved.
- Liver ultrasound. Single or multiple cysts are seen: aspiration of the cyst yields an "anchovy sauce"–like substance.

Etiology and pathogenesis

Amebic abscess is caused by *Entamoeba histolytica* that initially causes a diarrhea illness with subsequent spread via the portovenous system into the liver. The initial bowel infection may not be clinically apparent. Inflammation of the portal tracts and development of single or multiple abscesses follow.

Complications

Complications of amebic abscess include rupture of the cyst, causing peritonitis and secondary infection.

Prognosis

Patients with amebic abscess have a good overall prognosis if the condition is treated adequately.

Treatment

Metronidazole is the antibiotic of choice, given for 2 weeks. Diloxanide may be required to eradicate intestinal amebic cysts. Abscesses should be aspirated for diagnostic and therapeutic purposes.

Surgical drainage may be necessary in resistant cases or in the event of multiple large abscesses.

Parasitic infection of the liver

Hydatid disease
Incidence

Hydatid disease occurs worldwide but is more common where sheep and cattle farming are the main sources of living. Hydatid disease is rarely seen in the United States, and when seen, it is seen among immigrants from high-risk areas.

Clinical features

The clinical features of hydatid disease include the following:
- The disease is asymptomatic.
- The patient may experience right upper quadrant discomfort due to cystic enlargement and jaundice if obstruction of the bile duct occurs.
- Rupture in the abdominal cavity may cause fever, abdominal pain, and peritonitis.
- Hepatomegaly due to cystic formation can occur.
- Rupture of hydatid cyst into the biliary tree can cause cholangitis, biliary obstruction, and acute pancreatitis.

Diagnosis and evaluation

Appropriate tests include:
- Complete blood count. Peripheral eosinophilia is typically seen.
- Hemagglutination test. Results will be positive for hydatid disease.
- Liver biochemistry. Levels are normal unless obstruction of bile duct occurs, causing jaundice.
- Liver ultrasound. This will reveal cystic lesion with or without daughter cysts.
- Plain abdominal X-ray. This is not routinely done, but calcification of the cyst may be seen incidentally.

Etiology and pathogenesis

Hydatid disease is caused by ingestion of *Echinococcus granulosus* (a dog tapeworm) and its embryo via contaminated fruit and vegetables or direct ingestion due to poor hygiene (Fig. 18.31).

Within the duodenum, the embryos hatch and enter the portovenous system, and systemic spread to the lung, kidney, and brain can occur as well as to the liver.

Complications

Cyst rupture and secondary infection are the main complications. Rupture in the bronchus and renal tract may cause hemoptysis and hematuria, respectively. Brain cyst may present as epilepsy due to its space-occupying effects.

Prognosis

If adequately treated, complete recovery is expected.

Treatment

Treatment involves sterilization of the noncommunicating cyst (e.g., by injection of formalin or oral albendazole—can also reduce the size of cysts), followed by surgical resection of the intact cyst. Fine-needle aspiration is not routinely done due to risk of anaphylactic reaction to cyst contents.

Asymptomatic calcified cysts are usually left without treatment.

Prevention is undertaken by reducing carriage in domestic animals and improving hygiene.

Schistosomiasis
Incidence

Schistosomiasis is prevalent worldwide, affecting over 200 million persons, mainly in the tropics.

Clinical features

The main features of schistosomiasis are:
- Acute inflammatory response at the site of penetration through skin by the cercariae ("swimmer's itch").
- Fever, myalgia, malaise, GI upset (i.e., vomiting and diarrhea in the acute phase).
- Chronic infection producing hepatomegaly with or without portal hypertension.

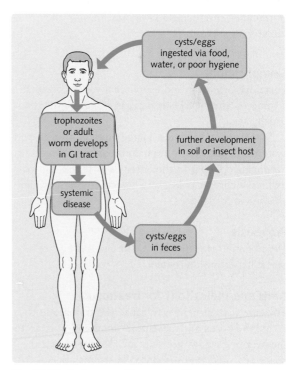

Fig. 18.31 Body map with parasitic life cycle.

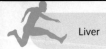

Diagnosis and evaluation

Tests of use include:

- Complete blood count. Watch for eosinophilia.
- Liver function test. Raised alkaline phosphatase level will be present with disease.
- Immunologic test. A positive result is not necessarily indicative of current infection because IgG antibodies remain after the disease has resolved.
- Detection of ova in stool, liver, or rectal biopsy specimens.

Etiology and pathogenesis

Schistosomiasis is predominantly caused by *Schistosoma mansoni* (Africa and South America) and *Schistosoma japonicum* (China and Southeast Asia). The mode of infection is via swimming or bathing in contaminated water, and its intermediate host is the snail.

The infective form of the parasite, cercaria, penetrates the skin and migrates via the portovenous system into the liver. Here, the parasite matures and eventually migrates along the portal and mesentric veins to produce a large amount of eggs, which leave the body by penetrating the intestinal wall to be excreted back into the river to complete its life cycle.

Granulomatous reaction to the trematode occurs in the liver, producing a periportal fibrosis and hepatomegaly.

Complications

Portal hypertension and esophageal varices occur in advanced cases of schistosomiasis, but cirrhosis is not usually seen.

S. japonicum produces a large number of eggs, and systemic deposition of ova in lungs or brain can occur, producing epilepsy in the latter case. It also causes extensive chronic colitis and can cause premalignant changes in some cases.

Prognosis

Despite adequate treatment, fibrosis and risk of portal hypertension remain.

Aims and indications for treatment

The aim of treatment is to cause the trematode to vacate the portal and mesenteric veins and migrate to the liver or lung, where they are destroyed by the host's cell-mediated response. There may be difficulty in curative treatment because the reinfection rate is high and it therefore may not be appropriate to attempt a cure.

Treatment

Praziquantel is an effective agent for all *Schistosoma* species. Abdominal pain and diarrhea are common shortly after the start of treatment.

Fascioliasis

Incidence

Fascioliasis is a zoonosis that infects sheep, cattle, and goats. It is transmitted to humans via contaminated vegetables. Fascioliasis occurs worldwide, including incidence in the United States.

Clinical features

Typical symptoms include:

- Fever, malaise, hepatomegaly, abdominal discomfort, and weight loss.
- Urticarial reaction due to migration of the parasite.
- Jaundice and cholangitis due to its presence in the biliary tract.

Diagnosis and evaluation

Tests to consider include:

- Full blood count. Watch for eosinophilia.
- Liver biochemistry. A cholestatic picture is seen.
- Serologic test. Specific complement fixation tests are now available.
- Duodenal aspiration. Ova are detected in stool in up to one third of cases.

Treatment

Bithionol or praziquantel is an effective treatment.

Polycystic liver syndromes

Polycystic liver disease includes many different disorders that have in common cystic lesions of the liver. Classification is difficult.

Incidence

The most important entity is adult polycystic liver disease, in which multiple cysts that do not usually communicate with the biliary tree develop in the liver. This condition is inherited as an autosomal dominant trait, and its incidence is approximately 1:5000 births. A related but less common condition is inherited as a recessive trait and often involves communication with the biliary tree.

Caroli's disease is a variant, comprising cystic dilatation of the biliary tree.

Congenital hepatic fibrosis is often included under the umbrella classification of polycystic liver disease because microcysts are common.

Polycystic liver disease is frequently associated with cyst formation elsewhere. Cysts are found in the kidney in 60% of cases and other viscera, especially the pancreas, in 5% of cases.

Clinical features

The clinical importance of these cysts (Fig. 18.32) is that they are often found incidentally during investigation for other problems and occasionally cause diagnostic confusion. Sometimes cysts present with pain, usually due to hemorrhage. Cysts related to the biliary tree or kidney can become infected.

Unless they are symptomatic in these respects, cysts of the liver or kidney do not usually present any problems. Cysts that communicate with the biliary tree are thought to have some malignant potential.

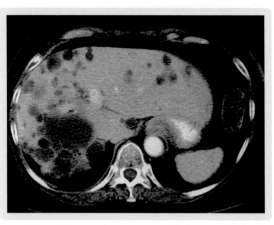

Fig. 18.32 CT scan of abdomen showing multiple cysts of different sizes in the liver.

Treatment

Because most cysts are asymptomatic, usually no treatment is indicated. Cysts causing hemorrhage or pain may require drainage, surgical fenestration, or resection. Superadded bacterial infection should be treated empirically to cover gram-negative organisms in particular. Cysts in the biliary tree occasionally require endoscopic drainage or resection.

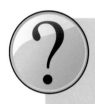

- Describe the functions of the liver under the subheadings of synthesis, storage, metabolic, and excretory.
- What are the clinical manifestations of an acute viral hepatitis?
- Describe the sequence of serologic markers and transaminases detected in the blood during acute hepatitis B infection (HBsAg, HBeAg, HBV DNA, ALT, anti-HBe, and anti-HBs antibodies).
- Name seven systemic manifestations of primary hemachromatosis in terms of end-organ damage.
- What are the clinical and biochemical parameters that comprise the modified Childs classification of cirrhosis?
- How would you manage a patient presenting with acetaminophen overdose? (Include clinical assessment, tests, and initial treatment strategy.)
- What are the factors associated with a poor prognosis in liver failure?
- Name some drugs known to cause disturbance in liver function.

19. Biliary Tract

Anatomy, physiology, and function of the hepatobiliary system

Bile canaliculi between hepatocytes form ductules that merge into bile ducts in the portal tracts. These ultimately form the right and left hepatic ducts, which leave the respective lobes of the liver and join together to form the common hepatic duct at the porta hepatis. The cystic duct from the gallbladder inserts into the lower end of the common hepatic duct to form the common bile duct, which courses through the head of pancreas to emerge in the second part of the duodenum together with the pancreatic duct (Fig. 19.1).

Bile consists of:

- Water.
- Bile acids. These are synthesized from cholesterol and act as a detergent for lipid stabilizers to form micelles with their hydrophilic and hydrophobic ends to enable absorption and digestion of fats.
- Cholesterol.
- Bilirubin. This is predominantly a by-product of the breakdown of red blood cells in Kupffer cells. Bilirubin is unconjugated and water-insoluble. Conjugation occurs in the liver to allow excretion with bile in the small duodenum. Once in the terminal ileum, bacterial enzymes deconjugate the molecule and a small proportion of free bilirubin (water-insoluble) is reduced to urobilinogen (water-soluble) and excreted as stercobilinogen in the stool. The rest is reabsorbed in the terminal ileum and into the liver via enterohepatic circulation and further excretion in bile. Urobilinogen can also be excreted via the kidneys (Fig. 19.2).

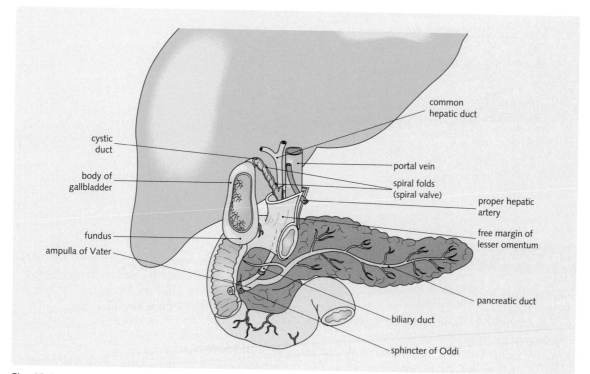

Fig. 19.1 Anatomy of the biliary tract and its relations.

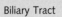

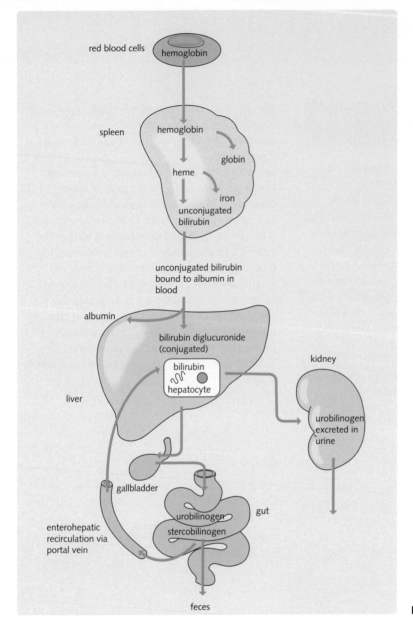

Fig. 19.2 Bilirubin metabolism.

Gallstones

It is important to distinguish between the following two conditions:
- "Cholelithiasis," which refers to the presence of gallstones in the gallbladder.
- "Choledocholithiasis," which refers to the clinical scenario whereupon the gallstone passes into the bile ducts.

Incidence
Gallstones can be found in approximately 30% of the population in the Western world in an age-related pattern (Fig. 19.3). They are rare in the Far East and Africa. Dietary factors may be influential.

Clinical features
Gallstones per se do not usually cause symptoms. More frequently, they are an incidental discovery

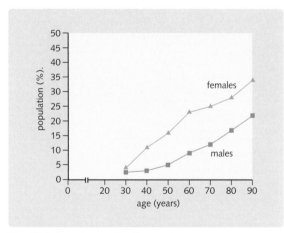

Fig. 19.3 Prevalence of gallstone disease.

during diagnostic imaging performed for another reason or are identified at autopsy. Symptoms such as flatulence, dyspepsia, and fat intolerance are commonly attributed to underlying gallstones, but whether there is a true correlation between the two is still debatable.

About 15% of patients with gallstones will require cholecystectomy for symptoms that may be attributable. The following symptoms and signs may occur:

- Biliary colic and cholecystitis account for over 90% of clinical presentations of gallstone disease.
- Cholangitis may occur if bile is infected; features include fever, right upper quadrant pain, and nausea and vomiting. Clinical jaundice is common. This is often seen in the presence of bile duct obstruction due to strictures or stones.
- Murphy's sign is elicited by placing two fingers on the right hypochondrium and asking the patient to breathe in. This results in pain and arrest of inspiration as the inflamed gallbladder moves below the costal margin. (It can be regarded as "positive" only if the same maneuver in the left upper quadrant does *not* cause pain.) Localized rebound and guarding are characteristic of cholecystitis.

Diagnosis and evaluation

A history of recurrent abdominal pain and jaundice with pale stools and dark urine, which subsequently resolves, may suggest an underlying diagnosis. Tests to confirm diagnosis should include:

- Complete blood count. Neutrophilia will be apparent if acute cholecystitis is present. Biliary colic alone can exist without superimposed infection.
- Biochemistry. Liver function tests may show features of obstructive jaundice (i.e., high bilirubin and alkaline phosphatase levels). Amylase levels should be checked to exclude acute pancreatitis, although they may be modestly raised in biliary colic or cholecystitis.
- Abdominal X-ray. This evaluation is not routinely done because only 10% of gallstones are radiopaque.
- Ultrasound. Although it is sensitive for the detection of gallstones, stones may not necessarily be the cause of clinical symptoms. Additional features, such as gallbladder wall thickening and tenderness over visualized gallbladder, are more diagnostic.
- Radioisotope scan. This test shows the function of the gallbladder and will demonstrate any blockages in the cystic or common bile duct by its delay in bile excretion (HIDA scan).
- Endoscopic retrograde cholangiopancreatography (ERCP) will show blockage in the common bile duct that may not be seen via ultrasound (Fig. 19.4).
- Endoluminal ultrasound and magnetic resonance cholangiography are useful alternatives to examine the bile duct without the risk of pancreatitis (see Fig. 24.20).

The diameter of the common bile duct should be less than 6 mm normally or less than 8 mm in a patient after cholecystectomy.

Etiology and pathogenesis

Three main types of gallstones have been described:

- Mixed stones constitute 70–90% of stones and predominantly contain cholesterol together with bile pigments and calcium. Multiple stones of different sizes are usually found, suggesting development in varying ages.
- Cholesterol stones account for up to 10% of stones and are usually solitary, smooth, and pale in color.
- Pigment stones, rare except in Asia, contain bile pigments (calcium bilirubinate) and are small and

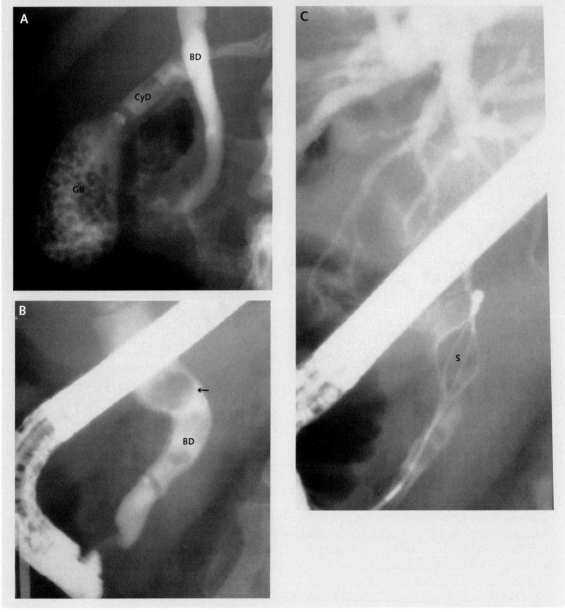

Fig. 19.4 Endoscopic retrograde cholangiopancreatography images. A. There are multiple small stones in the gallbladder (GB), but the bile duct (BD) is clear (CyD, cystic duct). B. A gallstone measuring 1 cm across can be seen in the middle of the common bile duct (arrow). C. A gallstone (S) in the bile duct is being retrieved with the grasping basket after sphincterotomy.

multiple. These are sometimes seen in patients with chronic hemolysis (e.g., hereditary spherocytosis, sickle cell disease) due to an increase in bile production.

The exact pathogenesis is unclear, although a high cholesterol intake and bile stasis have been implicated. There is usually a nidus of organic material, often containing bacteria, where precipitation of calcium and cholesterol takes place. This is enhanced by biliary stasis due either to infection or biliary obstruction.

Patients with terminal ileal disease are at an increased risk of developing gallstones. Because the terminal ileum is normally responsible for the resorption of bile salts, malfunction leads to a reduction of bile salts in the liver. Consequently, there is reduced micelle production and, hence, precipitation of cholesterol and formation of cholesterol stones.

Complications

In chronic cholecystitis, the gallbladder is shrunken and features of chronic inflammation are present. However, symptoms of intermittent abdominal pain, nausea, and vomiting can be due to other pathology. If recurrent, attacks of acute cholecystitis can give rise to chronic cholecystitis.

Empyema of the gallbladder means distention with pus, and the patient presents with a high, swinging pyrexia and septicemia. The risk of perforation and peritonitis is high.

Other complications include:

- Acute pancreatitis. Swelling or obstruction at the ampulla of Vater, secondary to gallstones in the common bile duct, is a common cause of acute pancreatitis.
- Ascending cholangitis. This can be the result of infection in the common bile duct spreading into intrahepatic ducts.
- Gallstone ileus. Erosion of the gallbladder wall by the stone can rarely cause peritonitis, and an ileus due to impaction of a large stone in the narrowed ileum can also occur.
- Carcinoma of the gallbladder. This is a rare complication.

Prognosis

Definitive surgery is usually curative, but occasionally in situ stone formation can occur in the common bile duct, causing recurrent symptoms.

Aims and indication for treatment

Asymptomatic patients require no treatment. Symptomatic patients can be treated either medically or surgically. Approximately only 15% of patients have symptoms over a 15-year period.

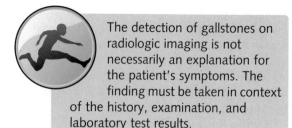

The detection of gallstones on radiologic imaging is not necessarily an explanation for the patient's symptoms. The finding must be taken in context of the history, examination, and laboratory test results.

Treatment

During acute episodes, if there are signs of infection, the following are required:

- Analgesia and antiemetics.
- Intravenous fluids.
- Blood culture tests, followed by the administration of broad-spectrum antibiotics.

Further intervention is not instituted at this stage unless perforation and generalized peritonitis occur.

Cholecystectomy, preferably laparoscopic, is often the treatment of choice, but some patients may not have the cardiorespiratory fitness for a general anesthetic.

ERCP is the treatment of choice for patients who have choledocholithiasis and have conditions unsuitable for surgery. An endoscope is inserted with the patient under sedation, and contrast is injected to show any stones in the bile duct and gallbladder. A sphincterotomy is usually performed to allow passage of further stones once the bile duct is free of obstruction (see Fig. 19.4).

Chenodeoxycholic acid and ursodeoxycholic acid are bile acids that can be taken orally and increase cholesterol solubility in bile. Treatment takes up to 6 months to complete, and recurrence occurs in over 50% of patients once treatment is stopped. This dissolution treatment is rarely used.

Tumors of the biliary tract

Carcinoma of the gallbladder
Incidence

Carcinoma of the gallbladder is predominantly a disease of elderly persons (older than 60 years) but may also occur in younger persons. There may be an association with preexisting gallstones, suggesting chronic inflammation as a carcinogenic influence. Gallbladder cancer accounts for less than 1% of all adenocarcinomas.

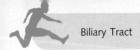

Clinical features

Jaundice, right upper quadrant mass, and general malaise and weight loss are common features. A number of cases are found incidentally on routine cholecystectomy and confirmed on histology.

Diagnosis and evaluations

Ultrasound is poor at detecting gallbladder carcinomas but will detect metastasis in the liver. The diagnosis is usually made at cholecystectomy for gallstone symptoms.

Prognosis

Due to the late presentation and early local metastasis of carcinoma of the gallbladder, patients rarely survive for more than 1 year.

Treatment

Radical resection of the tumor may provide a cure, especially for patients only diagnosed incidentally. Chemotherapy and radiotherapy have unproven benefits.

Cholangiocarcinoma
Incidence

Cholangiocarcinoma is an adenocarcinoma of the bile ducts associated with dense fibrous tissue. These tumors can be intrahepatic or extrahepatic. They are uncommon, accounting for only approximately 8–10% of primary liver tumors.

Clinical features

Features differ depending on the type of tumor:
- Extrahepatic tumors present with progressive jaundice similar to sclerosing cholangitis.
- Intrahepatic tumors tend to invade the liver parenchyma and present in a similar fashion to primary liver tumors, with jaundice being rare.

Clinical features such as weight loss, malaise, nausea, and vomiting may be evident.

Diagnosis and evaluation

Appropriate tests should include the following:
- Liver biochemistry indicates cholestatic jaundice with high alkaline phosphatase and bilirubin levels.
- Ultrasound, computed tomography, or magnetic resonance imaging shows dilated bile ducts if extrahepatic lesions are present, or lesions within the liver parenchyma if intrahepatic, but these

features are not specific for cholangiocarcinoma; therefore, ERCP is required.
- ERCP is also useful; the dense fibrous tumor tends to grow along the duct system, with the appearance of a shouldered stricture.

Etiology and pathogenesis

The etiology and pathogenesis of cholangiocarcinoma are unknown, but in the Far East there is an association with infestation by the fluke *Opisthorchis sinensis* (formerly identified as *Clonorchis sinensis*). Up to 20% of patients who have chronic symptomatic primary sclerosing cholangitis develop cholangiocarcinoma.

Chronic inflammation or sepsis may therefore be important etiologic factors.

Prognosis

The prognosis for cholangiocarcinoma is poor, with survival rarely lasting more than 6 months.

Treatment

Treatment options include the following:
- Radical resection of extrahepatic tumors can offer a cure, but this is rare.
- Insertion of endoprostheses (stents) during ERCP (see Fig. 24.18) will provide symptomatic relief of jaundice and improve quality of life.

Radiotherapy and chemotherapy are unhelpful treatment modalities.

Ampullary tumor

An ampullary tumor occurs when an adenocarcinoma arising from the ampulla of Vater presents with obstructive jaundice, which may be intermittent or progressive.

These tumors can be friable and bleed, presenting with melena or anemia with jaundice.

Diagnosis is made at ERCP, and if made early, tumors are amenable to resection with a 60% 5-year survival rate.

Fig. 19.5 shows the pattern of bile duct tumors.

Benign anatomic bile duct problems

Choledochal cyst and other anomalies

Congenital dilatations of the bile duct are known as "choledochal cysts." The majority are asymptomatic

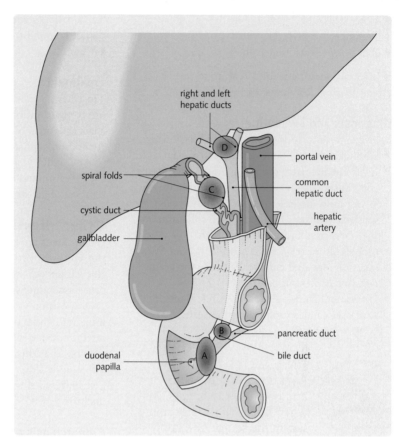

Fig. 19.5 Depiction of tumors involving the bile duct that may then present with jaundice. A. Ampullary tumor. B. Carcinoma of the head of the pancreas. C. Carcinoma of the cystic duct or gallbladder. D. Cholangiocarcinoma involving the hilum or below.

but can produce jaundice and abdominal pain. Intrahepatic cystic dilatations are known as "Caroli's disease" and can predispose the patient to cholangitis. Treatment of symptoms initiates with antibiotics, but surgical reconstruction may be required.

Benign stricture of the bile duct

Benign stricture of the bile duct is a result of damage to the bile ducts due to trauma or inflammation (e.g., gallstones, ascending cholangitis, or previous gallbladder surgery). It presents as progressive jaundice and can be mistaken for cholangiocarcinoma or sclerosing cholangitis.

Diagnosis is usually made by temporal association with trauma or surgery. Differentiation from tumors can be difficult if the trauma occurred a long time ago. Endoscopic brush cytology or histology may be helpful. Strictures occur in up to 15% patients after liver transplantation. Localized strictures can be treated with stenting or reconstruction surgery.

Infections of the biliary tract

Under normal circumstances, bile within the biliary tree is sterile. The sphincter of Oddi, together with hydrochloric acid in the gastric juice, prevents bacteria from ascending the tract.

Infection tends to occur only when the integrity of the bile duct sphincter function has been disrupted (e.g., after surgery or by inflammation caused by gallstones).

Cholangitis

Incidence

Cholangitis is a potentially serious but common complication of bile stasis that results from gallstones, bile duct dilatation, or strictures.

Clinical features

In the majority of persons with cholangitis, the symptoms are:

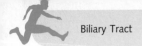

- Fever.
- Jaundice.
- Right upper quadrant pain.

Septicemic shock may be a feature in severe cases, especially in elderly persons.

Diagnosis and evaluation

Relevant tests to consider include the following:
- Complete blood count demonstrates neutrophilia.
- Liver biochemistry reveals a cholestatic picture (i.e., raised alkaline phosphatase and bilirubin levels, mild increase in transaminase levels). As a sensitive marker of infection and inflammation, the C-reactive protein level is high.
- Blood culture results are positive in over 90% of cases on repeated cultures (usually the gram-negative *Escherichia coli*).
- Ultrasound shows dilatation of bile ducts; liver abscesses can also sometimes be seen.

Always consider the biliary tract as a potential site of infection when faced with a patient in whom the source of (gram-negative) bacteremia is not obvious.

Etiology and pathogenesis

Cholangitis is commonly an *E. coli* infection resulting from bile stasis.

Causes include:
- Gallstones.
- Cholecystectomy (postsurgical).
- Benign strictures.
- ERCP (especially if a stent is inserted because stents occlude with time).

Complications

One related complication is suppurative cholangitis, a potentially fatal condition that requires urgent drainage either endoscopically or surgically. The diagnosis should particularly be considered in those patients whose fever and septicemic shock do not respond to appropriate intravenous antibiotics.

Treatment

Treatment consists of high-dose, broad-spectrum intravenous antibiotics to cover gram-negative and anaerobic organisms in particular (e.g., a third-generation cephalosporin and metronidazole).

Any underlying cause needs to be addressed once the infection has been adequately dealt with (e.g., removal of gallstones, blocked endoprosthesis).

Other infections of the biliary tract

Other infections of the biliary tract are rarely seen in the Western world and include infection with O. *sinensis* and C. *sinensis*, which are liver flukes that cause ascending cholangitis. There may be a predisposition to cholangiocarcinoma after such an infection. Patients with AIDS following HIV infection can develop sclerosing cholangitis, and it is possible that this could be due to opportunistic infection with *Cryptosporidium parvum* in the gastrointestinal tract, but its exact association is unclear.

Clonorchiasis and opisthorchiasis
Incidence

C. *sinensis* and O. *felineus* are common flukes found in the Far East that mainly affect animals such as dogs, cats, and pigs.

Clinical features

Patients with clonorchiasis or opisthorchiasis may remain symptom free, but repeated and prolonged exposure will cause:
- Recurrent jaundice.
- Cholangitis.
- Liver abscess.
- Possibly cholangiocarcinoma.

Diagnosis and evaluation

Microscopic examination of feces or duodenal aspirate is required for diagnosis of clonorchiasis or opisthorchiasis.

Treatment

Praziquantel is the treatment of choice.

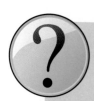

- What are the main constituents of bile?
- Describe the sequence of bilirubin metabolism and excretion.
- What are the clinical manifestations of gallstone disease, and what initial tests would you perform?
- How would you manage a patient presenting with symptoms and signs suggestive of acute cholecystitis?
- What is Murphy's sign?
- Why are patients with terminal ileal disease at increased risk of developing gallstones?

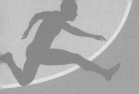

20. Pancreas

Anatomy, physiology, and function of the pancreas

The pancreas is a retroperitoneal structure that extends from the second part of the duodenum to the spleen (Fig. 20.1). The pancreatic duct, together with the common bile duct, enters the duodenum at the ampulla of Vater.

The pancreas has two distinct functions—exocrine and endocrine:

- Exocrine secretions include lipase, amylase, and proteases, which are responsible for digestion of fat, carbohydrate, and protein, respectively. The enzymatic secretion is influenced by gut hormones, such as cholecystokinin, which are released when fatty acids and amino acids enter the duodenum.
- Endocrine secretions are insulin, glucagon, and somatostatin; these hormones are primarily involved in the regulation of glucose storage and use.

Acute pancreatitis

Incidence
Acute pancreatitis is a relatively common condition affecting approximately 1% of the general population.

Clinical features
The clinical features of acute pancreatitis include:

- Severe epigastric pain that typically radiates to the back; sitting forward is sometimes said to provide some relief.
- Nausea and vomiting are invariably present.
- Tenderness and guarding, depending on severity.
- Tachycardia, tachypnea, fever, and shock may manifest in severe cases.
- Abdominal wall discoloration (i.e., bruising around the umbilicus [Cullen's sign] or over the flanks [Grey Turner's sign]). This is rare and reflects retroperitoneal hemorrhage that is likely due to a

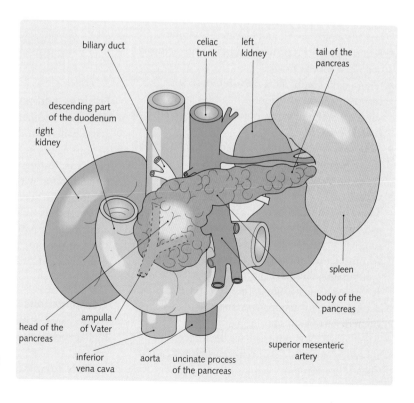

Fig. 20.1 The pancreas and related organs.

171

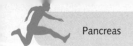
coagulopathy as a result of disseminated intravascular coagulation (DIC).

Beware of tachypnea in a patient with acute pancreatitis; this may be a reflection of severe metabolic acidosis or a manifestation of acute respiratory distress syndrome.

Diagnosis and evaluation

The tests performed should be as those for an acute abdomen because other conditions may mimic clinical signs and symptoms of acute pancreatitis.

In particular, consider the following tests:

- Serum amylase measurement. More than 1000 units is usually diagnostic. A lipase assay, although less readily available, has a longer half-life and a greater specificity.
- Biochemistry. A poor prognosis is associated with high glucose, high urea, low calcium, and low albumin levels (Fig. 20.2).
- Complete blood count and coagulation tests. Evidence of acute pancreatitis would include a high white blood cell count and evidence of DIC suggested by low platelet counts, high prothrombin time and activated partial thromboplastin time, low fibrinogen level, and elevated D-dimers.
- Arterial gases. Hypoxia with metabolic acidosis occurs in severe cases.
- Chest radiograph. This may demonstrate a reactive pleural effusion or bilateral infiltrates suggestive of acute respiratory distress syndrome (ARDS).
- Abdominal radiograph. The reported abdominal X-ray findings in acute pancreatitis are unreliable and not usually of diagnostic help.
- Ultrasound/computed tomography (CT) scans. These are routinely done. Swollen pancreas, ascites, and gallstones can be seen. Despite its unreliability in diagnostic terms, ultrasound is recommended initially in all patients with acute pancreatitis. An early diagnosis of gallstones in a severe case may prompt the need for endoscopic retrograde cholangiopancreatography (ERCP) to be undertaken.
- Many prognostic criteria have been recommended; however, none of these criteria replaces careful clinical assessment.

Poor prognostic criteria in pancreatitis	
Age	>55 years
White blood cell count	>15 × 10³/mL
Blood glucose	>200 mg/dL
BUN	>25 mg/dL
Albumin	<30 g/L
Calcium	<8 mg/dL
AST	>100 IU/L
LDH	>600 IU/L
PaO₂	<60 mmHg

Three or more of these factors indicate a poor prognosis (Glasgow scoring system)

Fig. 20.2 Prognostic criteria of severity in pancreatitis (BUN, blood urea nitrogen; AST, aspartate aminotransferase; LDH, lactate dehydrogenase; PaO$_2$, partial pressure of oxygen in arterial blood).

Modest elevations in serum amylase levels (usually <1000 IU) can be seen in a range of intra-abdominal conditions, such as acute cholecystitis, mesenteric infarction, and perforated peptic ulcer.

Etiology and pathogenesis

The exact mechanism of etiology and pathogenesis in acute pancreatitis is unclear, but is thought to be due to autodigestion by proteolytic enzymes in the pancreas, leading to self-perpetuating pancreatic inflammation with edema in mild cases and hemorrhagic necrosis in severe cases.

The reflux of bile in the pancreatic duct may contribute to pathogenesis of acute pancreatitis in cases of preexisting gallstones.

The causes of acute pancreatitis are listed in Fig. 20.3.

Complications

Acute pancreatitis is usually associated with a higher mortality rate, particularly if organ failure ensues.

Early complications include the following:

cysts are those occurring within the pancreas, and pseudocysts are those without an epithelial lining, consisting of a collection containing inflammatory fluid and pancreatic enzyme within the lesser sac. They are far more common than true cysts.

Multiple small cysts can also be seen in the pancreas with polycystic disease involving the kidney and liver. This is inherited as an autosomal dominant condition, and the pathology is quite different from that following acute pancreatitis; a more detailed text should be consulted for further information.

Clinical features

The main features of pseudocysts are as follows:
- Abdominal pain is present, particularly if the pseudocyst is large, together with nausea and vomiting mimicking unresolved acute pancreatitis.
- An epigastric mass may be palpable (the cyst will make the aorta more palpable and occasionally is mistaken for an aortic aneurysm).
- Ascites can occur due to rupture of the cyst within the peritoneal cavity. Ascitic fluid will have a high concentration of amylase.

Diagnosis and evaluation

The persistence or recurrence of symptoms after an episode of acute pancreatitis should alert one to the suspicion of pseudocyst formation (Fig. 20.5).

Ultrasound or CT scan is the test of choice, and small cysts are frequently seen in asymptomatic patients.

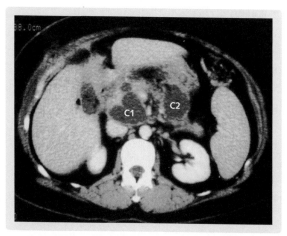

Fig. 20.5 CT scan of pancreatic pseudocyst. A heart-shaped cyst (C1) is seen in the head of the pancreas, and a second cyst (C2) is seen near the tail.

Etiology and pathogenesis

Pseudocysts are thought to be due to inflammatory exudate produced by the inflamed pancreas collected in the lesser sac. High levels of pancreatic enzyme found in the fluid may indicate extensive damage to the pancreas, causing secretions to leak out. They are more commonly found in severe and chronic pancreatitis.

Complications

Complications include pancreatic abscess, which is due to infection of the cyst that can occur spontaneously or as a consequence of repeated aspiration.

Prognosis

Prognosis depends on the underlying pathology. The expected outcome is poor if the pseudocyst is secondary to alcohol-induced chronic pancreatitis, whereas it is excellent if the pancreatitis is due to a treatable cause (e.g., gallstones).

Treatment

No treatment is required for small asymptomatic pseudocysts because they usually resolve spontaneously.

Therapeutic maneuvers include the following:
- Aspiration of a cyst is usually carried out under ultrasound guidance and may need to be repeated.
- Endoscopic drainage of a pseudocyst is being increasingly used these days. The drainage could be done with more precision with the help of endoscopic ultrasound.
- Surgery is recommended if the condition is persistent; the cyst can be "marsupialized" such that fluid will drain into the stomach.

Cystic fibrosis

Incidence

Cystic fibrosis affects 1 in 2500 live births.

Clinical features

The clinical features of cystic fibrosis include:
- Recurrent chest infections, usually the presenting feature in childhood.
- Pancreatic insufficiency leading to diabetes, steatorrhea, and failure to thrive despite a good appetite.

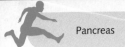

- Small bowel obstruction due to the viscous secretions. Neonates may present with meconium ileus.
- Infertility. Females are more likely to conceive; males are invariably infertile. Delayed puberty is seen in most patients with cystic fibrosis.
- Liver cirrhosis seen in patients who survive into adulthood.

Diagnosis and evaluation
Consider the following tests:
- Sweat test, which reveals a high sodium concentration.
- Genetic analysis for the recessive gene and the identification of cystic fibrosis protein.
- Pancreatic function tests (e.g., para-aminobenzoic acid [PABA] test).
- Chest radiography, which may demonstrate bronchiectatic changes. Spirometry and sputum culture should also be performed.

Etiology and pathogenesis
Cystic fibrosis is caused by a gene mutation on the long arm of chromosome 7 resulting in an abnormality of a transmembrane protein known as the "cystic fibrosis transmembrane conductance regulator," which results in production of thick viscous secretions (high in salt, low in water) due to reduced chloride transport.

Complications
The main complications of cystic fibrosis include malabsorption (especially of fat-soluble vitamins), bronchiectasis, and pneumothorax, which are common. Infertility and liver disease occur in adults. Death is usually due to respiratory failure.

Prognosis
The median survival is 30 years, with many affected adults in active employment. Persistent respiratory colonization with *Pseudomonas* organisms conveys a poorer prognosis.

Treatment
Treatment of chest infections includes intensive physiotherapy and appropriate antibiotic therapy. A recombinant nebulized DNAse aids in reducing sputum viscosity. Treatment can also include:
- Enzyme supplements (capsules containing trypsin and lipases, which break down in the duodenum delivering the enzyme).

- Immunizations.
- Vitamin supplements and a high calorie intake.
- Gene therapy. This has been attempted but early results are disappointing so far.
- Lung transplant, which is considered in some patients.

Carcinoma of the pancreas

Incidence
The incidence of carcinoma of the pancreas increases with increasing age, and most affected patients are older than 60 years of age. It is the fourth most common cancer in the United States, causing 32,000 deaths every year, and is more common in men than women.

Clinical features
Signs and symptoms include the following:
- Weight loss can be dramatic.
- Persistent abdominal pain is a common feature, usually radiating through to the back. This pain tends to be relieved by sitting forward.
- Jaundice is usually the presenting feature of carcinoma, affecting the head of the pancreas. Jaundice is obstructive and progressive and is characteristically painless in the early stages.
- Diabetes is thought to be due to insulin resistance caused by hormones secreted by pancreatic beta cells rather than its destruction.
- Thrombophlebitis migrans is a skin manifestation due to a paraneoplastic phenomenon.
- Ascites occurs in the late stages with hepatomegaly due to liver metastases.

Fig. 20.6 shows the sites at which pancreatic tumors occur.

 Courvoisier's law—in the case of painless obstructive jaundice, a palpable gallbladder suggests cancer because a dilated gallbladder is not found with gallstone disease as the stones induce a fibrotic reaction in the gallbladder, which then shrinks down.

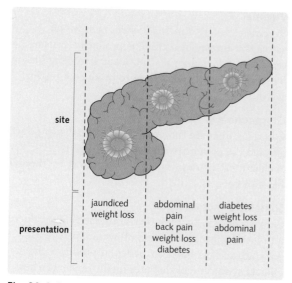

Fig. 20.6 Anatomic sites for pancreatic tumors.

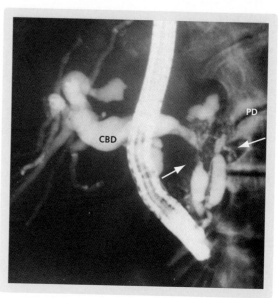

Fig. 20.7 ERCP scan showing "double duct stricture" (arrows) in pancreatic carcinoma (CBD, common bile duct; PD, pancreatic duct). Note incidental scoliosis and vertebral collapse.

Diagnosis and evaluation

Relevant tests may include the following:

- ERCP, as part of a test for obstructive jaundice, will usually be diagnostic—especially of periampullary tumors (Fig. 20.7).
- CT of the abdomen will diagnose most pancreatic tumors, and it is ideally confirmed by biopsy. It will also demonstrate nodal spread at the porta hepatis (Fig. 20.8).
- Ultrasound is less sensitive in detecting pancreatic tumors, especially those along the body or the tail of the pancreas.
- Endoscopic ultrasound is a major development in the diagnosis and staging of pancreatic cancer.

Etiology and pathogenesis

The etiology of carcinoma of the pancreas is unknown, but smoking and heavy alcohol consumption have been implicated. The role of chronic pancreatitis as a risk factor is uncertain because familial chronic pancreatitis is associated with a significantly increased risk of cancer.

Almost all tumors are due to adenocarcinoma arising from the duct epithelium, and approximately 70% are in the head of the pancreas. The tumors have usually already metastasized to local lymph nodes and the liver by the time of presentation.

Prognosis

The prognosis for carcinoma of the pancreas is very poor due to its late presentation. The 5-year survival rate is less than 5%.

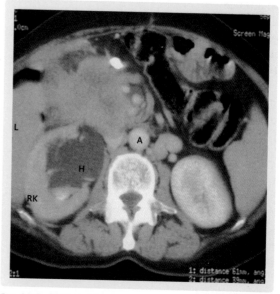

Fig. 20.8 CT scan of pancreatic tumor (arrows) obstructing the right ureter and causing hydronephrosis (H) (A, aorta; L, liver; RK, right kidney).

Aims of treatment

The aim of treatment is mainly for palliation because curative treatment is unlikely to be successful due to the nature of the disease.

Treatment

Treatment options include the following:

- Radical surgical resection provides the only possible chance of a cure, but it is seldom carried out because most patients are unsuitable for surgery and the surgery carries a high mortality rate. A bypass operation for the relief of jaundice can be performed in which the common bile duct is anastomosed to the small bowel as a palliative measure.
- Stent insertion can be achieved endoscopically; a stent is inserted into the narrowed part of the common bile duct to allow free drainage of bile (see Fig. 24.20).
- Analgesia in the form of opiates is indicated, as dependence is not an issue.
- Celiac axis block may be useful for patients with pain that is not controlled by conventional analgesia.

Endocrine tumors

Incidence

Endocrine tumors are rare in the pancreas and can occur with tumors of the pituitary and parathyroid to form a syndrome of multiple endocrine neoplasia (MEN).

Clinical features

Clinical features depend on the cell type and the hormone produced.

Gastrinomas (Zollinger-Ellison syndrome)

Gastrinomas arise from the G cells of the pancreas. They secrete gastrin and present as peptic ulceration, which is often large and multiple. Perforation and gastrointestinal hemorrhage are common, and the diagnosis should be considered in young patients presenting with recurrent peptic ulcer disease.

Diarrhea due to excess acid production is also common (low pH).

Insulinomas (islet cell tumors)

Insulinomas produce insulin and present as episodes of fasting hypoglycemia (i.e., early morning or late afternoon).

Presentation is often bizarre, hence diagnosis may not be made for years, and the patient learns to live with the symptoms because glucose abolishes the attacks.

Vipomas

Vipomas are rare pancreatic tumors in which vasoactive intestinal peptide is produced, causing severe secretory diarrhea and leading to dehydration by stimulating adenyl cyclase to produce intestinal secretions.

Glucagonomas

Glucagonomas are tumors of alpha cells that produce glucagon in patients with diabetes mellitus.

A characteristic rash (necrolytic migratory erythema) has also been described.

Somatostatinomas

Somatostatin is an inhibitory hormone that produces a reduction in the secretion of insulin, pancreatic enzyme, and bicarbonate; hence, it produces the clinical syndrome of diabetes mellitus, steatorrhea, and hypochlorhydria.

Weight loss is also a common feature.

Diagnosis and evaluation

The tests required for diagnosis are again dependent on the type of tumor involved and the clinical presentation:

- A CT scan and endoscopic ultrasound will identify the majority of endocrine tumors in the pancreas.

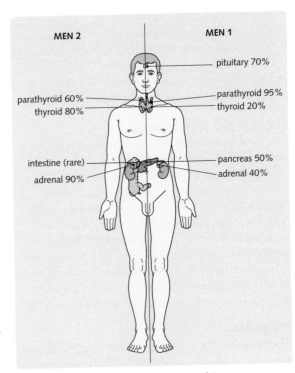

Fig. 20.9 Depiction of MEN types 1 and 2.

- Hormone assays measure the specific type of hormone produced and will often give the diagnosis. Selective venous sampling from the pancreas will also help to locate the tumor. In cases of insulinoma, measurement is usually made during a 24- to 48-hour fast when symptoms of hypoglycemia appear.

Etiology and pathogenesis

Endocrine tumors arise from the amine precursor uptake and decarboxylation cells, hence their hormonal secretory nature. The MEN type 2 syndrome has an autosomal dominant inheritance.

Prognosis

Gastrinomas are often malignant; therefore, they carry a worse prognosis than insulinoma, which is benign. The overall prognosis will depend on associated MEN syndrome and other tumors involved.

Treatment

Surgical resection of the tumor is required.

Identification of other possible tumors associated with MEN syndrome may be required, along with screening of relatives in those with MEN type 2 syndrome (Fig. 20.9).

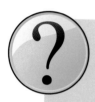

- Describe the functions of the pancreas.
- How would you manage a patient during the first few hours after an episode of acute pancreatitis?
- What are the factors indicating a poor outcome in the context of acute pancreatitis?
- What are the systemic complications of acute pancreatitis?
- What tests would you undertake in the investigation of suspected chronic pancreatitis?
- What is Courvoisier's law?
- What is the genetic abnormality described in cystic fibrosis?

HISTORY, EXAMINATION, AND COMMON INVESTIGATIONS

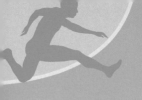

Preliminaries

Introduce yourself, be polite, listen carefully, and look interested, even if you have been up all night!

Give patients the time and the opportunity to tell you what you need to know and put them at their ease; many symptoms are embarrassing.

Try to maintain eye contact (even if patients do not), and watch carefully for clues to how ill they look. Are they agitated, distressed, or in pain? Is there a discernible tremor or involuntary movement? Is there evidence of significant weight loss (cachexia)? Do they have a pale, pigmented, or jaundiced complexion?

Look around the bedside for clues (e.g., inhalers, oxygen, a walking stick or frame, cards from family and friends, sputum pots, reading material and glasses, special food preparations).

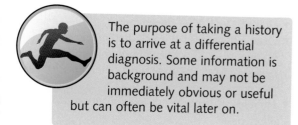

The purpose of taking a history is to arrive at a differential diagnosis. Some information is background and may not be immediately obvious or useful but can often be vital later on.

The standard structure of a history

It is important to maintain a structured approach to your history taking, particularly in the early stages of your career. You are less likely to omit relevant questions if your history is structured. It is preferable to commit the format to memory and to acquire the relevant information in conversational form, so that constant reference to notes is avoided during the interaction.

Description of the patient

This should include brief demographic details, including the patient's age, sex, ethnic origins, and occupation. It should allow others who have not met the patient to picture him or her in their mind.

Presenting complaint

What prompted the patient to seek help? This will usually be a specific or particular symptom but may be difficult to identify immediately. Your task is to focus on the symptoms and crystallize them into problems that can be addressed.

Note the sites of pain (Fig. 21.1).

History of the presenting complaint

This history of the presenting complaint is a complete description of the problem that brought the patient to see you, including:

- How and when the symptoms started.
- The speed of onset. Was it rapid, or slow and insidious?
- The pattern of symptoms and their duration and frequency. Are they continuous or intermittent? How often do they appear?
- If the symptoms include pain, a comprehensive description! Relevant features are onset, site, severity, character (e.g., sharp, crushing, gnawing), radiation, frequency, periodicity, associated features, precipitating and relieving factors, and relationship to meals, posture, and alcohol.
- The reason why the patient has decided to consult the doctor at this juncture. What is different?
- The extent of any deficit. Is there any loss of function, anything specific the patient cannot do, or any impact on lifestyle?
- Anything else the patient thinks may be relevant, however trivial.

Past medical history

Has the patient had any medical or surgical contact in the past? Ask specifically about operations, previous transfusions, use of drugs (especially antibiotics), allergies, and previous investigations.

Obstetric and menstrual history should also be recorded.

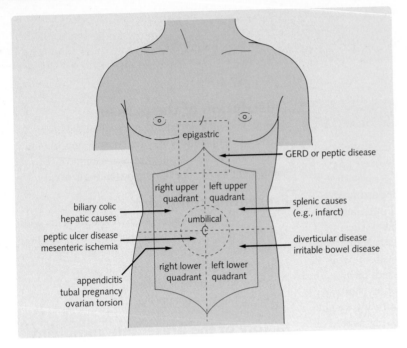

epigastric

GERD or peptic disease

right upper quadrant | left upper quadrant

biliary colic hepatic causes

umbilical

splenic causes (e.g., infarct)

peptic ulcer disease mesenteric ischemia

diverticular disease irritable bowel disease

right lower quadrant | left lower quadrant

appendicitis tubal pregnancy ovarian torsion

Fig. 21.1 Sites of pain and possible significance (GERD, gastroesophageal reflux disease).

Drug history

Ask about all drugs, including contraceptive pills and over-the-counter medicines as well as medicines that have been prescribed.

Nonsteroidal anti-inflammatory drugs are commonly taken as over-the-counter medicines and can cause ulcers.

It may be necessary to contact family members or the general practitioner to establish an accurate list of the patient's current prescribed therapy.

It is common for a patient to profess to have a drug allergy, when in fact an adverse side effect has occurred (e.g., diarrhea after taking penicillin or dyspepsia with aspirin). It is important to establish whether they are truly allergic to a particular drug because you may be denying them the best treatment. However, you must not prescribe anything to which they say they are allergic unless you are confident they are not!

Family history

Ask about the cause and age of death of close relatives, especially parents and siblings. Practice drawing quick sketches of family trees (Fig. 21.2). Is there a specific family history pertinent to the suspected diagnosis?

Social history

The purpose of this assessment is to see the patient in the context of his or her environment and to gain some idea of how the illness affects this particular patient, what support the patient has, and whether he or she can reduce any health risks.

It should include information about the patient's:
- Marital status.
- Children and other dependents.
- Occupational history (including previous occupations). This is especially relevant regarding exposure to toxins, musculoskeletal disorders, and psychiatry.
- Hobbies that may result in exposure to toxins or other risks.
- Accommodation. Put yourself in the patient's position: Will he or she be able to cope at home? Are there stairs, elevators, bath, shower, etc.?
- Diet. Is it adequate? High in cholesterol? Vegetarian?
- Exercise. Does he or she do any? Is it appropriate?

Is there any risk behavior?

Consider the following:
- Ask about alcohol use—record as units per day or week (Fig. 21.3).

- Ask about smoking—this is best described in terms of the number of "pack-years," whereby 20 cigarettes smoked each day for 1 year is termed "1 pack-year." (Forty cigarettes a day for 3 years would equate 6 pack-years.)
- Be tactful but thorough in asking about illicit or recreational drug use.
- Industrial toxins are important in claims for compensation (e.g., asbestos).
- A history of travel to certain regions of the world may be relevant.
- In addition to occupation or hobby, exposure to animals can be important.
- Sexual practice or orientation may be important for some conditions.

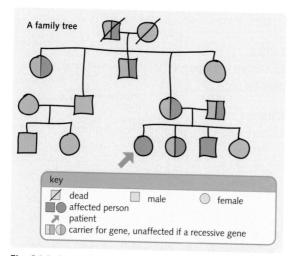

A family tree

key
- ▨ dead   ☐ male   ○ female
- ■● affected person
- ↗ patient
- ▧◖ carrier for gene, unaffected if a recessive gene

Fig. 21.2 Example of mendelian recessive inheritance depicted in a family tree. Arrow indicates the propositus, or individual who brought the pedigree to notice.

Review of systems (functional inquiry)

The purpose of this review is to go through the organ systems logically and ensure that nothing is forgotten. In addition, it often gives information into the cause or effect of the presenting complaint.

This can be very brief, and some of the important questions to ask are listed below. If the patient has any of these problems, clearly it is important to take a relevant extended history.

Gastrointestinal tract
Ask about:
- Abdominal pain.
- Indigestion.
- Nausea and vomiting.
- Heartburn.
- Dysphagia.
- Hematemesis and melena.
- Jaundice.
- Abdominal swelling.
- Change of bowel habit.
- Diarrhea.
- Rectal bleeding or pain.
- Weight loss.

(For a full discussion of these symptoms, refer to Part I.)

Cardiovascular system
Questions should include the following issues:
- Ask about chest pain related to exertion or posture.

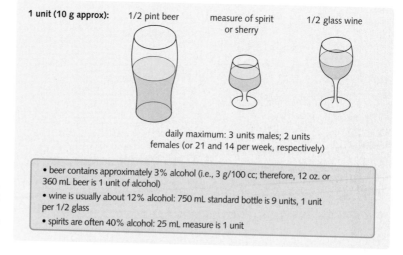

1 unit (10 g approx):   1/2 pint beer   measure of spirit or sherry   1/2 glass wine

daily maximum: 3 units males; 2 units females (or 21 and 14 per week, respectively)

- beer contains approximately 3% alcohol (i.e., 3 g/100 cc; therefore, 12 oz. or 360 mL beer is 1 unit of alcohol)
- wine is usually about 12% alcohol: 750 mL standard bottle is 9 units, 1 unit per 1/2 glass
- spirits are often 40% alcohol: 25 mL measure is 1 unit

Fig. 21.3 Alcohol measures and recommended limits. Try to work out the units of alcohol for yourself. One unit of alcohol is in fact 8 g, but when working out measures it is rounded upward to 10 g to simplify the calculations.

- Ask about chest pain relieved by rest.
- Are there any palpitations or postural syncopal attacks?
- Intermittent claudication is a sign of peripheral vascular disease. Ask patients how far they can walk before the pain comes on.
- Breathlessness can be a manifestation of cardiac disease.
- "Orthopnea" refers to the patient being breathless when lying flat. This is due to increased hydrostatic pressure in the lungs consequent upon left ventricular dysfunction. It is usually measured in terms of the number of pillows required for sleeping. However, it is important to clarify why the patient uses several pillows—it may just be for a bad back!
- Investigate symptoms of paroxysmal nocturnal dyspnea—the patient wakes up from the lying-down position gasping for air for reasons similar to those for orthopnea.

Respiratory system

Does the patient experience any chest pain? Is it "pleuritic," related to phases of respiration? Has there been any wheeze, cough, or hemoptysis? If there is sputum, inquire about color, nature, and amount.

Endocrine and reproductive systems

Has there been any:
- Polyuria or polydipsia (indicative of diabetes, hypercalcemia)?
- Heat or cold intolerance with mood change and/or weight change (suggestive of thyroid disease)?

- Fatigue with pigmentation and dizzy spells (possibly Addison's disease)?
- Erectile/fertility (male) or menstrual/fertility (female) problems?

Genitourinary tract

Is there any dysuria, nocturia, hesitancy, dribbling or incontinence, or urethral discharge?

Central nervous system

Inquire about any history of specific symptoms, such as:
- Headache.
- Speech or visual disturbance.
- Dizzy spells.
- Fits or blackouts.
- Loss of power or sensation in any area.

Joints

Has there been pain or swelling in any joint, or any back pain?

Skin

Is there a skin rash, itchiness (i.e., pruritus), or lumps or bumps?

Try to formulate an impression or differential diagnosis based on the history before proceeding to examination. You may be able to anticipate abnormal physical signs.

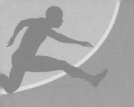

22. Examination of the Patient

The purpose of the clinical examination is to find evidence in support of or against the differential diagnosis you are considering after taking the history. It should be thorough enough so as not to miss other possibilities that you had not considered and to consider the causes and effects of each putative diagnosis.

Examination preliminaries

The main purpose of a general inspection is to determine how ill the patient is. Bear this in mind as you introduce yourself and take a history; if the patient is very ill, do not waste valuable time asking questions that can wait until later.

During the examination:
- Look at the patient's facial expression: Is he or she comfortable? In obvious distress? Looking furtive, receptive, or hostile?
- Assess the patient's body posture and mobility as well as weight and size.
- Consider whether he or she is appropriately dressed and behaving appropriately in the circumstances.

Many diseases and conditions do not have a direct effect on the gut. However, always remember that the patient may be receiving medication for a preexisting condition, and this may affect the dose of drug you are intending to give for his or her gastrointestinal (GI) condition (e.g., the patient may already be receiving enzyme-inducing drugs for another condition). Current medication may even be producing the gut symptoms (e.g., diarrhea caused by antibiotic therapy).

The following examination primer is orientated for GI disorders and is not comprehensive. You should read the *Crash Course* text relating to the relevant system to learn about other disorders.

Face

The face can be a mine of information. Some "facies" are pathognomonic of certain conditions (e.g., dystrophia myotonica, Graves' disease, and acromegaly) and have a peculiar habit of appearing in clinical examinations. Here, we concentrate on the facial signs of GI disease.

General inspection

Ask yourself the following questions:
- Are there any signs of mania or psychosis? (This might be related to steroids, systemic lupus erythematosus, Wilson's disease, or porphyria.)
- Is the patient agitated and not just anxious to see you? (This is a possible sign of hyperthyroidism, alcohol withdrawal.)
- Is the patient's general appearance unkempt or neglected (e.g., due to alcohol or depression)?
- Is there excessive skin hair? (Hypertrichosis can occur with excess steroids, cyclosporine, or minoxidil.)
- What is the skin's color and its relevance (Fig. 22.1)?

Are there specific skin lesions suggestive of a particular disorder (Fig. 22.2), such as:
- Dermatitis herpetiformis (celiac).
- Psoriasis (colitis, sometimes liver disease).
- Eczema (atopy).
- Telangiectasia (calcinosis cutis, Raynaud's phenomenon, esophageal stricture or dysmotility, scleroderma, telangiectasia [CREST syndrome]).

Pigmentation of the skin and its significance in gastroenterology	
Color	**Possible significance**
Yellow	Jaundice, carotenemia
Gray	Hemochromatosis
Brown	Addison's
Dusky	Primary biliary cirrhosis, renal failure
Blue	Cyanosis (cardiac, respiratory)
Red	Plethora, carcinoid flush
Blotchy	Vitiligo

Fig. 22.1 Pigmentation of the skin and its significance in gastroenterology.

- Spider nevi (liver disease).
- Erythema nodosum (inflammatory bowel disease, tuberculosis).
- Pyoderma gangrenosum (ulcerative colitis).

Specific examination

Examine the face specifically for particular signs indicative of disease (Fig. 22.3).

Hands

Examine the hands for particular signs indicative of GI-related disease (Figs 22.4 and 22.5).

Take the pulse, blood pressure, and feel the palms for temperature.

Find out whether there is:

- Any tremor: is it coarse or fine? Does it disappear with voluntary intent?
- A flap indicative of liver failure or carbon dioxide retention.

Neck, thorax, and upper limbs

Examine the neck and upper chest together looking for signs of:

- Liver disease.
- Portal hypertension.

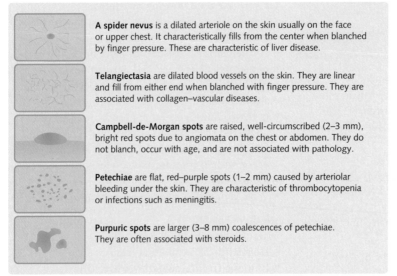

A spider nevus is a dilated arteriole on the skin usually on the face or upper chest. It characteristically fills from the center when blanched by finger pressure. These are characteristic of liver disease.

Telangiectasia are dilated blood vessels on the skin. They are linear and fill from either end when blanched with finger pressure. They are associated with collagen–vascular diseases.

Campbell-de-Morgan spots are raised, well-circumscribed (2–3 mm), bright red spots due to angiomata on the chest or abdomen. They do not blanch, occur with age, and are not associated with pathology.

Petechiae are flat, red–purple spots (1–2 mm) caused by arteriolar bleeding under the skin. They are characteristic of thrombocytopenia or infections such as meningitis.

Purpuric spots are larger (3–8 mm) coalescences of petechiae. They are often associated with steroids.

Fig. 22.2 Definitions of common skin lesions found in GI examination.

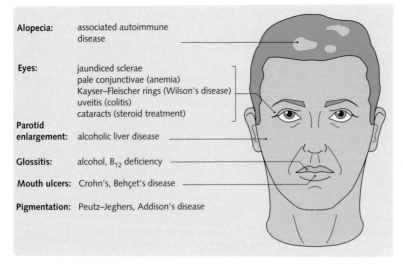

Alopecia: associated autoimmune disease

Eyes: jaundiced sclerae
pale conjunctivae (anemia)
Kayser–Fleischer rings (Wilson's disease)
uveitis (colitis)
cataracts (steroid treatment)

Parotid enlargement: alcoholic liver disease

Glossitis: alcohol, B_{12} deficiency

Mouth ulcers: Crohn's, Behçet's disease

Pigmentation: Peutz–Jeghers, Addison's disease

Fig. 22.3 Specific facial features of GI and liver disease.

Causes of abdominal masses		
Right iliac fossa mass	**Hepatomegaly**	**Splenomegaly**
Appendix abscess	Cirrhosis (PBC)	Portal hypertension
Ectopic pregnancy	Metastases/neoplasia	Myelofibrosis or CML
Crohn's mass	Hepatitis	Lymphoma
Ileocecal TB	Alcoholic liver disease	CMV or EBV
Ovarian tumor/tubal	Congestion	mononucleosis
pregnancy	(Budd–Chiari)	Anemia: sickle cell, PA
Carcinoma caecum	Storage disorders	Storage: Gaucher's
Carcinoid tumor	Riedel's lobe	
Amebic abscess		

Fig. 22.12 Causes of common abdominal masses (TB, tuberculosis; PBC, primary biliary cirrhosis; CML, chronic myeloid leukemia; CMV, cytomegalovirus; EBV, Epstein-Barr virus; PA, pernicious anemia).

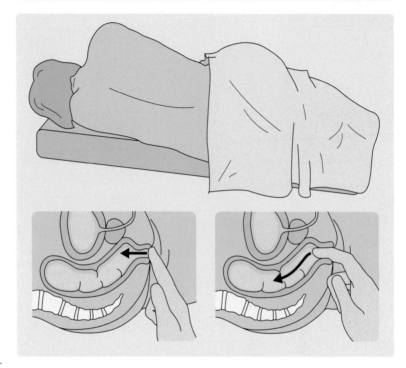

Fig. 22.13 Rectal examination technique: press gently on the anal margin with the pulp of your forefinger and gently rotate inward.

Causes of common abdominal masses are listed in Fig. 22.12.

 During superficial palpation for guarding and tenderness, be sure to look at the patient's face to check for reaction to pain.

Rectal examination

The rectal examination is a very important part of GI examination but must be carried out properly or is not worth doing. Clearly, there are sensitive issues of modesty and cultural code of which you need to be aware. Examination of a patient without consent may constitute an assault, and the more intimate examinations can be an area where failure to communicate your intention can produce difficulties.

Preparation

- Make sure the patient understands what you want to do and why (consent).
- Have a chaperone or assistant present (same sex as patient, if possible).
- Position the patient in the left lateral fetal position (bottom over the edge of the couch).
- Use lidocaine or K-Y Jelly on gloved hand.

Rectal examination technique

Inspect the anus for:
- Excoriation (pruritus ani).
- Tags (associated with colitis).
- External hemorrhoids.
- Fistulae (associated with Crohn's disease).

Press gently on the anal orifice with the pulp of your index fingertip and flex the finger through anal canal (Fig. 22.13). Gauge the sphincter tone: if necessary, ask the patient to squeeze.

Rotate your finger to feel the prostate or uterus anteriorly and the rectal mucosa all around, and assess the consistency of any stool present.

Look at the glove stain for blood or mucus.

Ancillary examinations are often available in the clinic to help with diagnosis.

These include:
- The guaiac test (Hemoccult) to examine the fecal stain for blood.
- Proctoscopy to examine the anal canal for fissures (painful) or hemorrhoids.
- Rigid or flexible sigmoidoscopy to inspect the rectal mucosa and take a biopsy specimen.

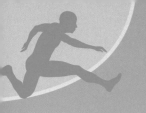

Purpose

The purpose of recording a history and examination in notes is to remind yourself and to convey to others what the patient's problems were at the time. Notes must be legible, timed or dated, and signed in order to be used by other professionals. Do not use abbreviations unless they are so well recognized as to be easily understood.

Be sure to remember **PDNUA**— **p**lease **d**o **n**ot **u**se **a**bbreviations!

Structure

Your history and notes will be much easier to follow if they are structured. Follow the same structure used in the history section of the sample medical history below. This is conventional and has the advantage that your colleagues will know where to look for specific information.

Illustration

Illustration can be very useful to document images or to convey very precisely the site of pain. Take care if you are using illustrations that, where they convey quantitative rather than qualitative data, they are clear (e.g., audible murmur 2/6, diminished muscle power 3/4). Examples are given in Figs. 23.1 through 23.4.

Formulating a differential diagnosis

It is important to convey your impression at the time of taking a history. The clinical picture may change later, but valuable clues can be gained by recording early impressions.

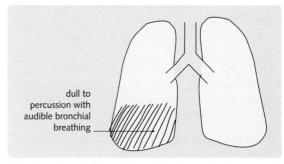

Fig. 23.1 Sample illustration of chest examination: usually the trachea and lung fields are drawn. The example shows an area of dullness to percussion, with audible bronchial breathing, in the lower right zone.

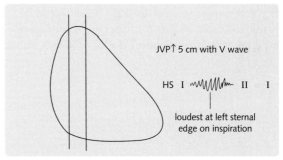

Fig. 23.2 Sample illustration of cardiac examination, showing how a murmur may be represented. In this example, a crescendo-diminuendo murmur was heard in systole (between the first and second heart sounds) and was best heard at the left sternal edge (JVP, jugular venous pressure; HS, heart sounds).

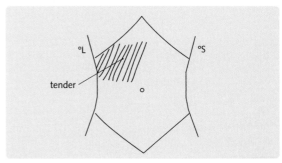

Fig. 23.3 Sample illustration of abdominal examination. In this example, there was an area of tenderness in the right upper quadrant. The degree symbol is often used to denote absence or negative findings (e.g., °L and °S indicate no hepatosplenomegaly found).

	Right arm	Left arm
Tone	↑	normal
Power	3/5	normal
Reflexes	++	+
Coordination	N/A (weak)	normal
Sensation	normal	normal

Fig. 23.4 Sample illustration of neurologic examination findings. Reflexes are often represented as present (+), brisk (++), or absent (−). The Medical Research Council scoring system for power should be used. Comments regarding type and distribution of sensory loss are made.

Investigation

If you are ordering investigations, these should be listed and dated so that it is clear when they were ordered. It is also very useful, if a list of investigations is required, that a summary of results is put alongside the list as it comes through.

Continuity

Clinical situations are rarely static. For subsequent entries, it is useful to state briefly the purpose or context of your review (e.g., called to see because complaining of chest pain).

If the clinical notes are extended because the patient has a long or complex history, a frequent update or summary is very useful to keep everyone focused on the problems. Some clinicians find it useful to keep a problem list that is updated daily. The important element throughout is clarity of thought and intent.

Sample medical history

An example of a medical history is shown in Fig. 23.5. It highlights some of the points discussed earlier in this chapter.

disease). It is more reliable, specific, and sensitive than a test of the erythrocyte sedimentation rate.

Biochemistry

Urea and electrolyte measurements are requested routinely for the majority of patients. Sodium levels are commonly slightly low in many sick patients due to the syndrome of inappropriate antidiuretic hormone secretion. Some inference about GI tract pathology can be made from routine biochemistry (Fig. 24.3).

Amylase

Some common features of amylase levels include the following:
- Should be at least moderately raised (500 IU/L) in acute pancreatitis.
- Are usually normal in the presence of chronic pancreatitis.
- Are commonly raised without pain after endoscopic retrograde cholangiopancreatography (ERCP).

Routine biochemistry		
Parameter	Level	GI significance
Urea	Low	Malabsorption or liver disease
	High	Slightly (up to 40 mg/dL): dehydration (nausea, vomiting, Addison's) Moderate (up to 60 mg/dL): profound dehydration, GI bleed (protein load) Severe (more than 60 mg/dL): renal failure, hepatorenal syndrome
Sodium (Na)	Low	Common in diarrhea, vomiting, alcoholic liver disease, diuretics
Potassium (K)	Low	Common in diarrhea, vomiting, alcoholic liver disease, loop diuretics
	High	Possible renal failure, diuretics especially spironolactone
Calcium (Ca)	Low	Correct for albumin, common in celiac disease
	High	Associated with malignant disease, hyperparathyroidism
Magnesium (Mg)	Low	Commonly in malnutrition, malabsorption, alcoholic diseases
Creatinine	High	Renal failure (all causes)
Glucose	High	Hyperglycemia can cause abdominal pain, dehydration, acidosis Acute and chronic pancreatitis can lead to high glucose in serum

Fig. 24.3 Routine biochemistry and its significance in GI disease.

- Are raised nonspecifically in many causes of abdominal pain (e.g., perforated viscus, ruptured ectopic pregnancy, cholecystitis).

Arterial blood gases

Patients who are ill from any cause (e.g., sepsis, liver/renal failure, pancreatitis) develop metabolic acidosis, often with compensatory respiratory alkalosis (hyperventilation). After an acetaminophen overdose, pH is a particularly useful prognostic measurement (along with the serum creatinine and prothrombin time).

Glucose

Diabetes mellitus can present in a spectrum of guises, including weight loss. Glucose measurement is often forgotten.

Calcium

Hypercalcemia can lead to constipation, and low levels can be seen in malabsorption and vitamin D deficiency.

Alcohol

Alcohol measurement can be useful in specific circumstances, such as determining occult causes of coma or abnormal liver enzymes in patients presenting acutely.

Endocrine and metabolic

Thyroid function

Thyroid disease does not usually cause GI tract problems but may accentuate symptoms such as diarrhea (hyperthyroidism) or constipation (hypothyroidism) from other causes. Hyperthyroidism needs to be excluded as a cause of weight loss. (In children, it can cause weight gain!)

Catecholamine levels

A 24-hour urinary collection for free catecholamines (i.e., epinephrine, norepinephrine, and dopamine) is used to diagnose catecholamine excess resulting from tumors of the adrenal medulla. These may present with GI symptoms of weight loss, nausea, vomiting, and altered bowel habit. Associated features are flushing and cardiovascular dysfunction (arrhythmias and episodic hypertension).

Cortisol

An absent or impaired cortisol response after the administration of an analog of adrenocorticotropic hormone is useful to diagnose Addison's disease. This can present with nausea, vomiting, weight loss, diarrhea, or postural dizziness. Acute adrenal failure may present as severe abdominal pain, mimicking an acute abdomen.

Gut hormone profile

Serum gastrin

Serum gastrin levels are raised slightly in patients with *Helicobacter pylori* infection or peptic ulcer disease and in patients receiving long-term treatment with proton pump inhibitors. They are markedly raised in cases of gastrinomas. These amine precursor uptake and decarboxylation (APUD) tumors arise most commonly in the pancreas but also in the mucosa of the duodenum or antrum. They present with peptic ulcers, diarrhea, and weight loss.

Urinary 5-hydroxyindoleacetic acid

5-Hydroxyindoleacetic acid is a breakdown product of 5-hydroxytryptamine (serotonin, 5-HT) produced by argentaffin cells. Primary carcinoid tumors arise in the small intestine or rectum. The clinical syndrome of 5-HT excess only occurs when there are liver metastases, as "first-pass" hepatic metabolism is avoided. It involves abdominal pain and watery diarrhea. Associated features are facial flushing and respiratory wheeze.

Vasoactive intestinal peptide

Vasoactive intestinal peptide is produced in excess by rare pancreatic tumors and causes severe watery diarrhea.

Glucagon

Glucagon is produced in excess by alpha cell tumors of the pancreas, resulting in diabetes mellitus and a characteristic skin rash.

Somatostatinomas

Somatostatinomas produce diarrhea and weight loss with diabetes mellitus.

Porphyrins

Porphyrins are intermediate metabolites in the heme biosynthetic pathway. Enzyme absence or deficiency in the pathway results in their accumulation, leading to:

- Neuropsychiatric disorder.
- Hypertension.
- Photosensitive skin rashes.

GI presentation is common with abdominal pain, vomiting, and constipation. Excess porphobilinogen is found in urine. Red blood cell porphobilinogen deaminase and aminolevulinic acid synthase, the most common enzyme deficiencies, can be measured (Fig. 24.4).

Nutrient elements

Iron

Serum iron is subject to too much fluctuation to be useful on its own. When compared with its binding capacity (total iron binding capacity), the percentage saturation of transferrin can be derived:

- Values below 20% are considered to depict iron deficiency.
- Values above 50% probably indicate iron overload.

(See Chapter 11.)

When saturation levels are borderline abnormal, repeat the test with the patient in a fasting state.

Ferritin

Ferritin reflects body iron stores in adults and is a useful tool for investigating iron overload. However, as an acute-phase protein, its levels are elevated in

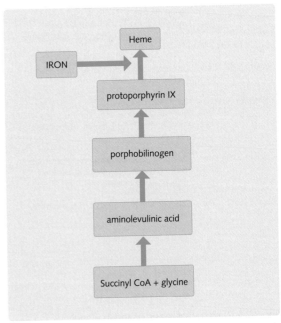

Fig. 24.4 Heme biosynthetic pathway (CoA, coenzyme A).

any cause of inflammation. It can therefore be misleadingly normal or high in rheumatoid arthritis or in alcoholic hepatitis, in which cases it may be difficult to differentiate from hemochromatosis.

Ceruloplasmin

A plasma protein that binds copper, ceruloplasmin is reduced in most cases of Wilson's disease, but this is not sufficient to make a diagnosis. Serum copper levels should also be elevated and 24-hour urinary copper excretion increased.

Zinc

Zinc levels are low in alcoholic and other chronic liver diseases; its deficiency can cause an enteropathy as well as skin rashes.

Liver enzymes and liver function tests

Liver enzymes

Elevated liver enzyme levels in serum signify hepatic injury of some kind but give no information about liver function. For this, routine measurement of metabolites made or excreted by the liver are very useful (e.g., bilirubin, albumin, coagulant factors). Dynamic function tests are also available, although rarely used.

Use Figs. 24.5 and 24.6 to help you to work out how to interpret liver enzyme levels.

The pattern of elevation may give some clue about the disease process. This is easiest to understand by reference to the hepatic lobule in Fig. 24.6:

- A predominant or disproportionate rise in alkaline phosphatase and gamma glutamyl transferase levels indicates biliary tract pathology such as obstruction or biliary cirrhosis.
- A predominant rise in transaminase levels usually indicates a parenchymal process such as hepatitis.

Tests of liver function
Standard blood tests

Prothrombin time is a sensitive test of hepatic synthetic function because it reflects interaction of all the clotting factors made by the liver (II, VII, IX, and X). It is often expressed as international normalized ratio (INR) against a control.

In cholestatic syndromes, prothrombin time may also be abnormal because absent bile reduces absorption of vitamin K from the intestine. In this situation, the INR will correct with parenteral vitamin K but not in parenchymal liver disease. Be aware that parenteral vitamin K will take at least 6 hours to become effective. Albumin depletes rapidly in chronic debilitating or inflammatory conditions. It is made in the liver (half-life, 20 days) and is low in chronic liver disease and malabsorption. It can also fall in the acute setting, such as severe sepsis or an acute inflammatory condition.

Bilirubin levels in serum can be conjugated or unconjugated:

- Unconjugated elevation (clinically referred to as "acholuric jaundice") occurs in hemolytic disorders or with deficiencies of conjugation enzyme (e.g., Gilbert's disease, Rotor's syndrome).
- Conjugated hyperbilirubinemia indicates cholestasis or loss of hepatocyte function.

Elevation of liver enzymes	
Liver enzymes	**Significance**
AST (aspartate transaminase)	Very high (thousands) in acute hepatitis or necrosis Moderate (approx. 500) in chronic active inflammatory disease Mild (<300) in portal tract damage, focal hepatitis Also present in muscle (raised in myocardial infarction)
ALT (alanine transaminase)	As for AST, but more specific to liver In alcoholic hepatitis usually less than AST by ratio of 2
Alkaline phosphatase	Highest in cholestatic syndromes (portal tract disease or bile duct obstruction). Remember other sources: bones (especially young), placenta (females), intestine (rare)
Gamma glutamyl transferase	Very labile enzyme, often mildly elevated Highest levels in portal tract disease and alcoholics

Fig. 24.5 Elevation of liver enzymes and their significance.

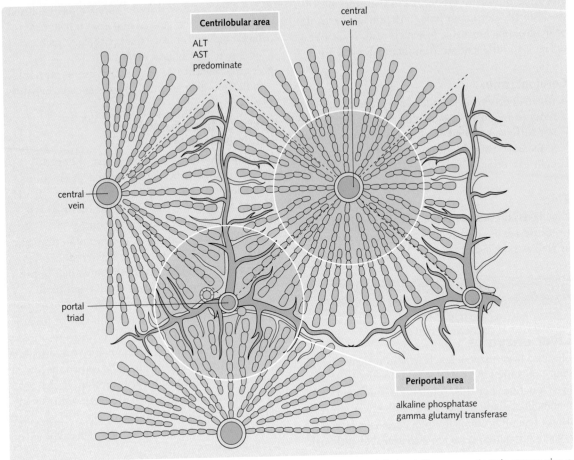

Fig. 24.6 Liver enzymes predominate in different areas of the liver lobule, and their relative proportions in serum give a clue about the pathologic process in the liver (ALT, alanine transaminase; AST, aspartate transaminase).

Prothrombin time can be prolonged because of poor synthesis of clotting factors in liver disease and will not be corrected by vitamin K. Alternatively, it may be prolonged due to a lack of vitamin K absorption because of biliary obstruction. In this instance, parenteral vitamin K can be expected to correct the prothrombin time.

Causes of jaundice include (see Chapter 12):
- Hepatitis (viral and alcoholic).
- Drugs (e.g., phenothiazines, anticonvulsants, some antibiotics such as clavulanic acid and flucloxacillin).
- Poisons (e.g., carbon tetrachloride, CCl_4).
- Chronic liver diseases such as primary biliary cirrhosis or primary sclerosing cholangitis.
- Extrahepatic bile duct obstruction (e.g., gallstones and benign or malignant bile duct strictures).

It is often forgotten that gluconeogenesis and glycogenolysis (the mechanisms for the homoeostasis of blood glucose levels) take place in the liver.

Profound hypoglycemia can occur in some acute liver diseases (e.g., fulminant hepatic failure, Reye's syndrome) and occasionally with alcoholic binges. Glucose tolerance is impaired in chronic liver diseases.

Immunoglobulins are commonly elevated in chronic liver disease but not usually in obstructive jaundice or in drug-induced cholestasis.

The mechanisms of elevation are poorly understood, however:

- In cirrhosis, this may involve antigens from the gut bypassing the liver and producing an antibody response predominantly of immunoglobulin (Ig) G and IgM classes.
- In alcoholic liver disease, a decline in Kupffer cell activity may explain the rise in IgA levels because of reduced clearance.
- High IgG levels are usually associated with chronic active hepatitis and IgM with primary biliary cirrhosis.

Dynamic and metabolic liver tests

Dynamic and metabolic liver tests are based on the principle that certain substances are either metabolized or excreted by the liver and their products can be measured after administration as a bolus (Fig. 24.7).

These tests are mainly useful as research tools and for evaluating response to new treatments. Some of the more commonly used tests are described briefly below.

Sulfobromophalein sodium excretion

Sulfobromophalein sodium (BSP) is an organic anion that is rapidly taken up by the liver and bound by Y and Z proteins before being excreted. A test for this excretion can detect subtle changes in hepatic dysfunction in cases of mild disease but is not often used clinically. Changes in serum albumin and hepatic blood flow affect the result. Delayed excretion is pathognomonic of Dubin-Johnson syndrome.

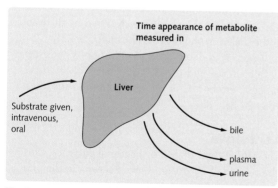

Fig. 24.7 Principle of dynamic liver function tests: a known amount of substrate is given and its metabolite(s) measured at set time points in plasma or urine. Metabolism is a function of hepatic functional mass and blood flow.

Indocyanine green

Indocyanine green is another organic anion that is more avidly bound to plasma protein and more actively extracted by the liver. It is safer, easier to measure, and less susceptible to variability than BSP but is less useful in detecting subtle changes in function. It reflects hepatic blood flow very well and is mostly used for this purpose. It is normal in Dubin-Johnson syndrome.

Bile acids

Bile acids more specifically reflect excretory hepatic function than serum bilirubin. They are sensitive and specific and can be used to detect subtle dysfunction or to differentiate liver disease from congenital hyperbilirubinemias or hemolysis. In practice, their measurement offers little advantage over enzyme estimation in combination with measurements of protein and bilirubin.

Iminodiacetic acid excretion (HIDA, DISIDA scans)

Iminodiacetic acid (IDA) derivatives are taken up by hepatocytes and excreted in bile. They can be tagged with a radioactive isotope (e.g., technetium-99) to evaluate excretory function and gallbladder concentration of bile. They can be useful in difficult cases of intrahepatic bile duct stasis.

Metabolic challenge tests

Metabolic challenge tests rely on functional hepatic mass to produce or excrete a metabolite.

Antipyrine clearance, aminopyrine breath test, and caffeine or lidocaine clearance have been used to investigate and test microsomal function. They correlate well with hepatic dysfunction but offer little advantage over the measurement of prothrombin time, serum albumin level, or the Child-Pugh score.

Galactose tolerance test

Galactose is rapidly phosphorylated in hepatocytes and eliminated. After an infusion or bolus, the rate of elimination can detect subclinical cirrhosis and distinguish parenchymal from obstructive liver disease. It offers no clinical advantage over orthodox tests.

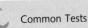

Liver biopsy

Ultimately, for a detailed assessment of liver pathology, a liver biopsy will often be required.

The usual indications are to help in diagnosis or to assess the severity of inflammation and fibrosis in established disease to guide treatment and prognosis.

The procedure is undertaken with or without ultrasound guidance, usually with a slicing or suction needle inserted percutaneously and with local anesthetic. A Menghini hollow, wide-bore needle inserted into the liver with suction via a syringe may be used as an alternative.

Subcostal or shoulder tip pain (diaphragmatic referred pain) is common. More serious complications include bile leak or hemorrhage. Perforation of a viscus is rare (mortality, 1:1000).

If coagulation is abnormal (a 4-second prolongation of prothrombin time) or there is significant thrombocytopenia (80,000), a biopsy specimen can be obtained with a long, flexible needle via the jugular and hepatic veins or by laparoscopy under direct vision. The standard vital stains used are hematoxylin and eosin and reticulin to demonstrate fibrosis.

Tests of pancreatic and gastric function

These tests are now rarely used, and for the majority, the sensitivity and specificity are too poor to be relied on.

Pentagastrin
The gastric acid output is measured preceding and following the administration of pentagastrin (a synthetic gastrin analog).
- High basal output results from high gastrin levels (now known to be due to *H. pylori* infection) or very high levels (in Zollinger-Ellison syndrome).
- A low maximal output response indicates atrophic gastritis or achlorhydria.

Lundh test
After a fatty meal, duodenal content is aspirated and assayed for trypsin and lipase. The levels are low in chronic pancreatitis. Variations of this test are also undertaken with secretin or cholecystokinin provocation.

Para-aminobenzoic acid
Para-aminobenzoic acid (PABA) is a peptide hydrolyzed by chymotrypsin, causing release of free PABA, which is excreted in the urine. A less than expected amount of PABA in the urine after an oral load is diagnostic of pancreatic insufficiency.

Fat malabsorption
Fat malabsorption can be determined by detecting a high proportion of unabsorbed fat after a test meal (3-day fecal fat collection) or detecting a lower than expected amount of $^{14}CO_2$ in exhaled air after an oral dose of ^{14}C-labeled triglyceride (e.g., ^{14}C triolein). To confirm that this result is due to pancreatic insufficiency, it is often compared and expressed as a ratio to $^{14}CO_2$ after an oral dose of fatty acid (e.g., ^{14}C oleic acid).

Pancreolauryl test
Fluorescein-conjugated dilaurate is hydrolyzed by pancreatic esterase; the released fluorescein is absorbed and detectable in urine. False-positive results may occur if bacterial esterases are present.

Breath tests

The general principle of breath tests is that a substrate is metabolized when the relevant enzyme is present in the gut lumen, resulting in release of CO_2 or hydrogen, which are absorbed by diffusion and exhaled in the breath. Normally, breath hydrogen is undetectable, so elevation is consistent with bacterial hydrolysis. To detect CO_2 by this process, either ^{13}C or ^{14}C is used in the substrate (Fig. 24.8).

Lactulose
Lactulose is hydrolyzed by bacterial enzymes, causing the release of hydrogen. Once bacteria in the oral cavity are neutralized with an antiseptic mouthwash, an early rise will indicate bacteria in the proximal small intestine beyond the stomach. A late rise, due to bacteria resident in the colon, is normal.

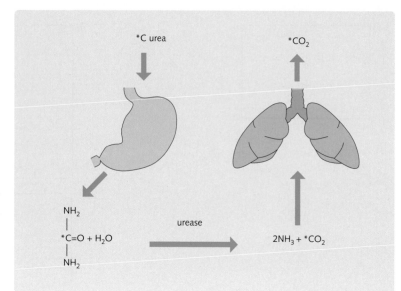

Fig. 24.8 Schematic representation of the biochemical basis of gut breath tests. The example shown is the urea breath test in which ^{13}C or ^{14}C urea is given orally. If urease is present in the stomach (on the cell membrane of *H. pylori*), the urea is split into ammonia and radiolabeled CO_2, which can be detected in the exhaled breath. *C indicates that C is radiolabeled.

Lactose

Lactose is cleaved by disaccharidase, allowing its constituent sugars to be absorbed. Failure to detect a rise of plasma glucose after an oral load of lactose indicates disaccharidase deficiency, which can be congenital or due to any small bowel disorder. Avoidance of dairy products usually alleviates the associated diarrhea.

d-Xylose

d-Xylose is a synthetic sugar absorbed, like all sugars, from the proximal small intestine. Measurement of serum xylose after an oral load has been used as a test for malabsorption but is too sensitive and nonspecific to be clinically useful.

Urea

Urea labeled with ^{13}C or ^{14}C and given orally is cleaved to ammonia and radiolabeled CO_2, which is detectable in exhaled breath if urease is present in the stomach. This enzyme is present on the coat of *H. pylori*, and the test identifies patients with current gastric infection.

Glycolic acid

Glycolic acid is a bile salt that can be conjugated to ^{14}C glycine. Bacteria, if present in the small intestine, deconjugate the bile salt and the glycine is metabolized, releasing $^{14}CO_2$ which is absorbed and exhaled in expiration.

Motility physiology

Esophageal manometry

Esophageal manometry is undertaken for the investigation of noncardiac chest pain if esophageal dysmotility is suspected and in the assessment of gastroesophageal reflux disease or nonmechanical dysphagia.

A tube with either solid-state or water-pressure transducers at intervals along its length is passed nasogastrically, and peristaltic swallow waves are recorded (Figs. 24.9 and 24.10).

- Uncoordinated peristalsis with failure of the lower esophageal sphincter to relax is diagnostic of achalasia.
- High pressure waves (i.e., nutcracker esophagus) may indicate esophageal spasm.
- Diffuse hypomotility is common in scleroderma.

Ambulatory esophagogastric pH

Ambulatory esophagogastric pH testing is often undertaken in combination with manometry in the assessment and management of reflux disease. The patient wears the tube attached to a small solid-state recorder for 24 hours and the result is then analyzed by a computer (Figs. 24.11 and 24.12).

The transducer is placed 5 cm above the gastroesophageal junction, where the pH is normally

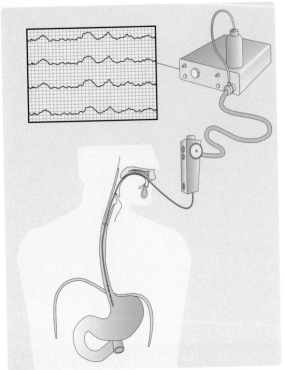

Fig. 24.9 Measurement of esophageal motility. A probe is passed nasogastrically with several transducers at 1-cm intervals. These pick up sequential pressure waves as the peristaltic swallow travels down the esophagus. This is represented by the waveforms shown in Fig. 24.10.

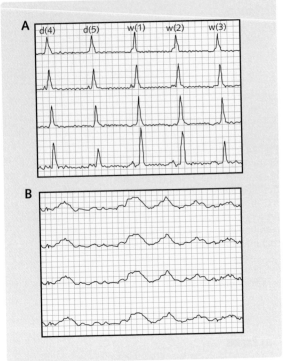

Fig. 24.10 Esophageal motility showing (A) normal peristalsis and (B) peristalsis from a patient with achalasia, in whom the peristalsis is uncoordinated. The lower sphincter also fails to relax in achalasia (not shown in this tracing).

above 4, and detects reflux of acid when the pH drops below 4. Results are expressed as the number of reflux episodes and the proportion of time that esophageal pH is below 4 (normally <5%).

Anorectal manometry

Anorectal manometry is undertaken for the investigation of fecal incontinence or chronic constipation. A narrow tube with pressure transducers is passed across the anus and measures resting tone and squeeze-relaxation activity. An inflatable balloon device attached to a pressure gauge is used to assess rectal pressures. The patient can be instructed by a biofeedback mechanism to improve anal sphincter tone and defecation technique.

Serologic tests

A large variety of tests are based on the interaction of antibodies with antigen in radioimmunoassay kits and enzyme-linked immunosorbent assay kits (Fig. 24.13). Their principal use is to screen for infection, tumors, or immunoinflammatory disease when those conditions are suspected because of the clinical presentation or the results of other tests.

These are useful confirmatory tests but are much less useful and often confusing if used as screening tests. Here they are classified according to their clinical implications in GI tract pathology.

Markers of autoimmune disease

Antibodies to various nuclear components are found in a number of diseases (Fig. 24.14) but also in up to 20% of the normal population.

More specific antibodies to double-stranded DNA are found in 50% of patients with systemic lupus erythematosus and speckled-pattern antinuclear factor in mixed connective tissue disease.

- Smooth muscle antibodies are found in 60% of cases of autoimmune chronic active hepatitis. Anti–liver-kidney microsomal antibodies are found in a subgroup of these patients.

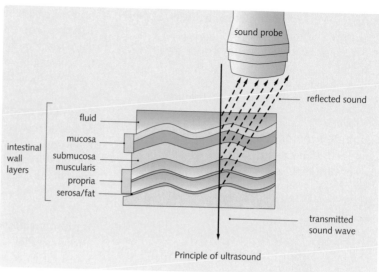

Fig. 24.19 Principle of ultrasound. A sound probe transmits an energy wave through the tissue. At the interface between layers of different density, some sound waves are reflected (echoed) back and can be translated into an image as shown in Fig. 24.20. Ultrasound probes can be used transcutaneously (transabdominal), endoscopically, or even endovascularly.

- Assessing anorectal damage (usually as a result of parturition or forceps delivery).
- Obtaining tissue diagnosis using fine-needle aspiration.

Endoluminal ultrasound is becoming increasingly important for the investigation of pancreatic abnormalities and tumors.

Bile duct manometry

Bile duct manometry is undertaken by passing a pressure transducer on a catheter through an ERCP endoscope. This is undertaken for rare causes of biliary pain thought to be due to biliary dyskinesia.

In this procedure, pressure waves are obtained as they are for esophageal manometry.

Laparoscopy

Laparoscopy is now increasingly undertaken to perform surgical operations such as cholecystectomy. However, the original and still very useful indication is for inspection of intra-abdominal organs, including the liver. Ultrasound and biopsy can also be undertaken through the laparoscope.

Radiology
Chest radiograph

A chest X-ray is useful in the investigation of liver disorders to assess heart size and concomitant pulmonary disease. In the investigation of patients with an acute abdomen, it is essential to look for evidence of air under the diaphragm on an erect film because this indicates a perforated intra-abdominal

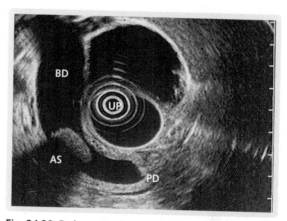

Fig. 24.20 Endoscopic ultrasound scan demonstrating a gallstone within the bile duct. An acoustic "shadow" (AS) is cast behind the stone. Note the ultrasound probe (UP), bile duct (BD), and pancreatic duct (PD).

viscus (see Fig. 3.1). Conversely, absence of a gastric air bubble can be a feature of achalasia.

Plain abdominal radiograph

Plain abdominal radiography is useful in suspected cases of obstruction to look for dilated bowel loops and fluid levels in the bowel (see Fig. 3.2). It is also useful in patients with colitis to assess mucosal edema and colonic dilatation.

Abdominal ultrasound

Abdominal ultrasound is undertaken in the investigation of abdominal pain (usually to exclude gallstones) or abnormal liver enzyme levels. It is useful in:

- Assessing bile duct dilatation, but it is only 60% sensitive in finding a cause.
- Screening for hepatic metastases or pancreatic tumors.
- Identifying ascites.
- Looking for occult gynecologic tumors.

Computed tomography

Computed tomography (CT) is an important investigative tool for gastroenterology. It is the primary means of staging all intra-abdominal tumors. It is the most sensitive noninvasive technique for diagnosing chronic pancreatitis. It can be useful for CT-colography as an alternative to barium enema or colonoscopy in the elderly.

Magnetic resonance

Magnetic resonance can differentiate different tissue characteristics without using radiation. With computer reconstruction, it is a sensitive technique to examine the bile duct or pancreas as an alternative to ERCP.

Barium swallow

Barium swallow is frequently undertaken in the investigation or assessment of dysphagia. Compared with endoscopy:

- The additional advantage of barium swallow is that peristaltic pressure waves are observed and signs of gastroesophageal reflux can be sought.
- The disadvantage is that direct inspection of the mucosa cannot be undertaken and biopsy specimens cannot be obtained.

Cine esophagogram

Cine esophagogram is similar to barium swallow except that the entire process of swallowing is visualized on fluoroscopy and recorded on video. This provides better information than static radiographs from traditional barium swallow, especially in the case of motility disorders.

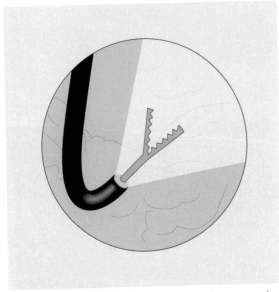

Fig. 24.21 Endoscopic biopsy—a grasping forceps can be used through the endoscope to obtain pinch biopsy specimens of mucosa.

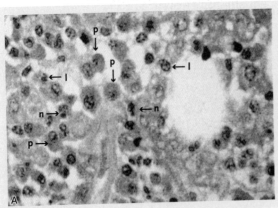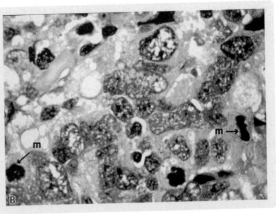

Fig. 24.22 Histologic examination is important for identifying the cause of inflammation or for demonstrating malignant transformation in tissue. A. Acute and chronic inflammation with neutrophils (n), plasma cells (p), lymphocytes (l), and the occasional eosinophil. B. Large pleomorphic (bizarrely shaped) nuclei with little cytoplasm (increased nuclear-cytoplasmic ratio). Mitotic (m) figures can be seen.